Handbook of
PHLEBOTOMY

GARLAND E. PENDERGRAPH, Ph.D.

*Director, Client Relations and Education,
and Laboratory Director for Satellite Laboratories
Doctors Laboratory, Inc.
Valdosta, Georgia*

THIRD EDITION

D0966438

Lea & Febiger • *Philadelphia* • *London* • *1992*

Lea & Febiger
200 Chester Field Parkway
Malvern, Pennsylvania 19355-9725
U.S.A.
(215) 251-2230

Executive Editor — Darlene Cooke
Project/Manuscript Editor — Dorothy Di Rienzi
Production Manager — Samuel A. Rondinelli

Library of Congress Cataloging-in-Publication Data

Pendergraph, Garland E.
  Handbook of phlebotomy / Garland E. Pendergraph. — 3rd ed.
  p.   cm.
  Includes bibliographical references and index
  ISBN 0-8121-1564-3
  1. Phlebotomy—Handbooks, manuals, etc. I. Title
  [DNLM: 1. Bloodletting—handbooks.   WB 39 P397h]
RB45.15.P46 1992
616.07′561—dc20
DNLM/DLC
for Library of Congress   91-46514
                                                              CIP

First Edition, 1984
Reprinted, 1985
Second Edition, 1988
Third Edition, 1992

PRINTED IN THE UNITED STATES OF AMERICA
Print number: 5 4 3 2 1

To the laboratory's envoys to the outside world: the phlebotomists

and

To the employees of Doctors Laboratory, Inc., who have made my life so enjoyable and my work such a pleasure

PREFACE

When I was in medical technology training, about the only things that concerned those doing venipunctures were to be sure that the burrs on the needles were not too terribly painful, and that the plungers were not frozen in the glass syringes because someone put them together before they were dry. Since those days a great many changes have taken place, and today our knowledge regarding proper specimen collection is far more sophisticated.

This book in no way pretends to be a definitive work on the subject of phlebotomy. It is, for the most part, directed toward the student phlebotomist and student laboratory technician or technologist. It attempts in a basic format to cover those procedures most likely to be done in a general health care institution. The step-by-step design is intended to make the procedures easier for the student to understand and follow. Also, the material is suitable for use by laboratory supervisors in the preparation of phlebotomy procedure manuals. Although the procedures outlined in this book are similar to those done in many laboratories, it must be remembered that some testing procedures have more than one correct methodology. Finally, it is important to remember that this book is only an outline or reference—a handbook. It can never replace the guiding hand of the patient and knowledgeable teacher.

Changes in this edition have been numerous. Many of the chapters have been revised, and the chapters on isolation technique and selected reference values have been deleted. Taking their places is the chapter on infection prevention and an appendix that gives several sources for teaching materials plus information on certifying organizations. Several of the illustrations have been upgraded and a few new ones have been added.

There are many to whom I am eternally grateful. First I wish once again to express my appreciation to all those individuals who helped me with the first two editions. Without their help and patience this edition would never have been. I especially want to thank Helen Maxwell, CPT(ASPT), not only for her support, but also for her many helpful suggestions and for sending me the information on phlebotomy certifying agencies used in the appendix. I wish to thank Patti Garcia, MT(ASCP), Bill McGehee, MT(ASCP), James Certa, C(ASCP), and David Williams, Ph.D. for their review of and suggestions for several of the chapters. To Karen Kennedy, CPT(ASPT) and Joni McCully, CPT(ASPT) who assisted me in making the new photographs on venipuncture technique and tourniquet application, I am most appreciative.

My appreciation also to those companies that allowed me to illustrate their products in Chapter 7. My thanks to the staff of Lea & Febiger for all the assistance they have given me. I especially want to remember Mr. Christian Spahr, Jr., whose guidance and encouragement will never be forgotten. He was my editor for the first and second editions and for this edition until his death on August 6, 1991. A special thank you to those who offered suggestions and constructive criticism regarding the previous editions. A number of the changes in this edition are a result of their help. I again solicit readers' suggestions. All mistakes or oversights in this book are my fault alone, and I accept full responsibility.

Nashville, Georgia   Garland E. Pendergraph

CONTENTS

Chapter
1. A Brief History of Phlebotomy 1
2. Professionalism 7
3. General Rules for Safety 10
4. Infection Prevention 13
      Biosafety Techniques 14
      Universal Precautions and Body Substance Isolation 14
      Handwashing 15
      Gowning, Gloving, and Masking 17
5. Medical Terms and Abbreviations 22
      Prefixes, Suffixes, and Word Roots 23
      Words and Terms 24
      General Abbreviations 31
      Often Used Clinical Laboratory Abbreviations 33
      Symbols 35
      Commonly Ordered Laboratory Tests 35
6. How the Heart and Circulation Work 38
      The Composition of Blood 38
      The Heart 41
      Veins and Arteries 45
      Basic Coagulation 48
7. The Blood Collection System 52
      Diagrams of Equipment 52
      How the Primary Anticoagulants Work 62
      Rubber Stopper Color Coding 63
      Primary Anticoagulants and Their Action 64
      Other Additives and Their Action 64
      Trouble Shooting and the Evacuated Blood Collection System 65
      Safety Devices 67
      Tube and Holder Size 68
8. Performance of a Routine Venipuncture 71
9. Procedure for a Skin Puncture 82
10. Nursery Technique 86
11. Arterial Punctures 87
12. Procedure When Unable to Obtain a Blood Specimen 90
      Patient Not in Room 90
      Patient Refuses to Allow Venipuncture 90

        Difficult Venipuncture 91
13.   Preparation of a Blood Smear 92
        The Coverslip Procedure 92
        The Slide-Wedge Procedure 93
14.   General Procedure for the UNOPETTE Brand Hematology System   97
15.   Special Collection Techniques 102
        Crossmatches 102
        Blood Cultures 104
        Oral Glucose Tolerance Test (GTT) 106
        Cold Agglutinins 109
        Fibrin Degradation Products 109
        Bleeding Time 110
        Heparin Lock Procedure 113
16.   General Collection Requirements 115
Appendix 119
Index 123

Chapter 1

A BRIEF HISTORY OF PHLEBOTOMY

An interesting fact about the history of phlebotomy is the lack of history about phlebotomy, insofar as the "letting" of blood for diagnostic rather than therapeutic purposes. The "letting" of blood for "healing" purposes has been practiced since antiquity, and practically every civilization has recorded its use. Phlebotomy was used as a therapeutic measure in the United States well into the eighteenth century.

Little is known about when blood was first used to diagnose disease. A bit more is known about the origin of the instruments of phlebotomy as they pertain to attaining blood for analysis. The familiar piston-and-cylinder syringe was first used on wounds as a "pus-puller." Its precise birth record is lost, but the concept of the piston and cylinder is attributed to the ingenuity of Ktesibios, the son of a barber in Alexandria, Egypt, around 280 BC. Its use to extract pus from wounds as well as another possible use—as a flame thrower—never caught on. This great instrument (an early example is illustrated in Figure 1-1) has been used during most of its existence for the injection of liquids.

When blood first began to be examined for diagnostic purposes is unknown although it is known that another body fluid, urine, has been examined since medieval times. The invention of the microscope in the seventeenth century, coupled with advancements in physiologic chemistry and cellular physiology in the nineteenth, paved the way for the examination of blood as a diagnostic tool, probably in the latter part of the nineteenth century.

It was not until 1908 that the first Manual of Clinical Diagnosis was published. The author was James C. Todd, a professor of clinical pathology at the University of Colorado School of Medicine. In the chapter The Blood, in the 1912 edition, is a sentence that will amuse most laboratorians. It reads: "For most clinical examinations only one drop of blood is required." The Manual, in addition to describing general techniques for obtaining blood by venipuncture and skin stick, discussed the latest laboratory procedures. A few of the important ones included the cigarette-paper (Zig-zag brand)

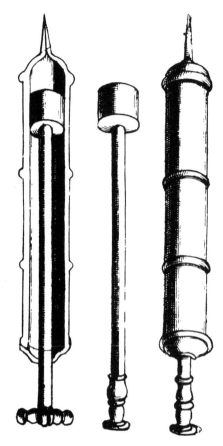

Fig. 1-1. An early piston-and-cylinder syringe. (From Majno, G.: The Healing Hand: Man and Wound in the Ancient World. Cambridge, Harvard University Press, 1975.)

method for making differential slides; fixing differential slides before staining by soaking in pure methyl alcohol for 15 minutes or heating in an oven at 150°C; and obtaining a blood culture from a skin puncture in the lobe of the ear. "By gentle milking, 20 to 40 drops can usually be obtained."

A few of the instruments that were recommended in early editions for use in obtaining blood are illustrated in Figures 1-2 through 1-4. Although the instrumentation recommended may appear somewhat crude as compared with the instrumentation of today, the concepts remain similar.

Little change occurred in either instrumentation or concepts until 1943, when an evacuated blood collection system, known as the VACUTAINER Brand, had its beginning. This system is discussed in more detail in Chapter 7. This was not the first evacuated system. The Keidel vacuum tube for the collection of blood was manufactured by Hynson, Wescott and Dunning, Baltimore, Maryland, around 1922. This system consisted of a sealed ampule with or without culture medium. Connected to the ampule was a short rubber tube with a needle at the end (Fig. 1-5). A small glass tube served as a cap.

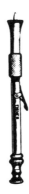

Fig. 1-2. Army-type blood lancet. (From Todd, J. C. et al.: Clinical Diagnosis by Laboratory Methods, 12th Ed. Philadelphia, W. B. Saunders, 1953.)

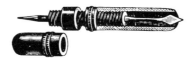

Fig. 1-3. Daland's blood lancet. (From Todd, J. C.: Clinical Diagnosis by Laboratory Methods, 5th Ed. Philadelphia, W. B. Saunders, 1923.)

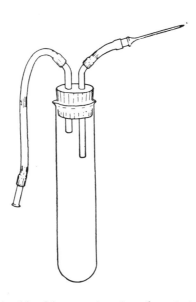

Fig. 1-4. A device for drawing blood from a vein using a large test tube. (From Todd, J. C. et al.: Clinical Diagnosis by Laboratory Methods, 8th Ed. Philadelphia, W. B. Saunders, 1937.)

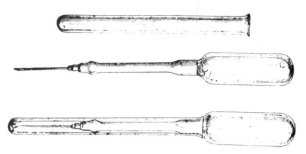

Fig. 1-5. Keidel's vacuum tube. (Todd, J. C. et al.: **Clinical Diagnosis by Laboratory Methods,** 8th Ed. Philadelphia, W. B. Saunders, 1937.)

After the needle had been inserted into the vein, the stem of the ampule was crushed. The blood entered the ampule because of the vacuum. For some reason this concept did not become popular until the VACUTAINER Brand. I own a Keidel vacuum tube with culture medium that was manufactured in 1922. The culture medium is still sterile.

With the introduction of the VACUTAINER Brand and similar evacuated blood collection systems came a new interest in improving techniques and reconsidering concepts related to phlebotomy. Great strides have been made since the days of manually sharpened needles with their ever-present and painful "burrs." Not only are needles now smaller and sharper, and skin lancets properly sterilized and less painful, but newer concepts of obtaining blood better assure more accurate results and less permanent damage to the patient.

There are two phlebotomy national organizations—the National Phlebotomy Association (NPA) (1978) and the American Society of Phlebotomy Technicians (ASPT) (1983). Certifying examinations are administered by NPA, ASPT, the National Certification Agency for Medical Laboratory Personnel, and the American Society of Clinical Pathologists.

What the future holds for phlebotomy is unknown, and to forecast would be foolhardy. It can be said without fear of contradiction, however, that the numerous scientific improvements and changes in philosophy reflect the efforts and contributions of many individuals who realize that obtaining a blood sample is much more than just a "sideline" to the other things we do in the laboratory.

No history of phlebotomy is complete without mentioning the history of circulation. The identity of the first person to recognize the importance of veins and arteries is lost with antiquity; however, as long ago as 2650 BC, Hwang-Ti, Emperor of China, made the observation that "all blood is under the control of the heart. The blood flows continuously in a circle and never stops." Even Hippocrates (ca. 460 to 380 BC), the father of medicine, noted: "The vessels spread themselves over the body filling it with spirit, juice, and motion are all of them but branches of an original vessel. I protest I know not where it begins or where it ends, for in a circle there is neither a beginning nor an end."

It would be another 2000 years before the correct movement of blood from the heart and its return to it would be outlined. Praxagoras of Cos (ca.

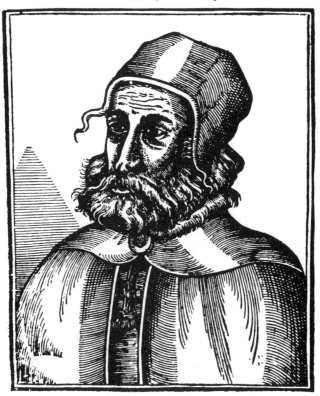

Fig. 1-6. Galen, ca. 130-200 AD. (From Haggard, H. W.: Devils, Drugs and Doctors. New York, Harper and Row, 1929.)

340 BC) was among the first to separate the functions of arteries and veins, but believed that both systems contained air. It was Galen (ca. 130 to 200 AD) (Fig. 1-6), an egotistical Greek physician from Pergamon, who showed that arteries are filled with blood, not air, which was still the prevalent thinking of the time. He also showed, with fair accuracy, the heart movements. But he did not stop there; he went on to theorize that the blood moved from the right side of the heart to the left through pores in the walls between the ventricles. This was but one of many of his anatomic mistakes.

That little or no knowledge was contributed about the circulation of blood for centuries after Galen's death testifies to his dictatorship over medicine until the critics of the Renaissance toppled him. For approximately the next 1500 years, men bowed to authority. Since the church had embraced the writings of Galen as the absolute truth, to propose other hypotheses contrary to Galen's teachings would be heresy. Many a man of science was slowly burned at the stake for doing so.

From time to time, there was a flicker of light. Around 1531, Michael Servetus maintained that the blood passed from one side of the heart to the other through the lungs. For his discovery of pulmonic circulation, he was rewarded by having his books confiscated and being burned at the stake.

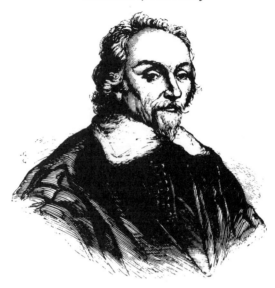

Fig. 1-7. Harvey, 1578-1657. (From Russell, J. R.: History and Heroes of the Art of Medicine. London, John Murray, 1861.)

In 1628, William Harvey (Fig. 1-7), in a lecture before the Fellows of the Royal College of Physicians, followed the passage of blood from the heart, through the arteries, to the veins, and back to the heart again. It was as if Hwang-Ti, that Emperor of China, had been his mentor. Actually, it was his anatomy professor, Fabricius of Aquapendente, and his work on the valves of the veins that gave stimulus to Harvey's conclusions.

How the blood passed from the arteries into the veins remained a mystery until around 1660 when Marcello Malpighi, the leading microscopist of his time, demonstrated capillary circulation.

BIBLIOGRAPHY

1. Haggard, H. W.: Devils, Drugs and Doctors. New York, Harper and Row, 1929.
2. Heath-Hammond, L. R., and Gelinas, C. E.: A history of phlebotomy in 18th-century America. Lab. Med., *13:*776, 1982.
3. Majno, G.: The Healing Hand: Man and Wound in the Ancient World. Cambridge, Harvard University Press, 1975.
4. Neuburger, M.: History of Medicine. Vol. I. Oxford, Oxford University Press, 1910.
5. Poynter, F. N. L., and Keele, K. D.: A Short History of Medicine. London, Mills and Boon, 1961.
6. Robinson, V.: The Story of Medicine. New York, Tudor Publishing, 1931.
7. Todd, J. C.: Clinical Diagnosis by Laboratory Methods, 2nd Ed. Philadelphia, W. B. Saunders, 1912.
8. Todd, J. C.: Clinical Diagnosis by Laboratory Methods, 5th Ed. Philadelphia, W. B. Saunders, 1923.
9. Todd, J. C., Sanford, A. H., and Wells, B. B.: Clinical Diagnosis by Laboratory Methods, 12th Ed. Philadelphia, W. B. Saunders, 1953.
10. Walker, K.: The Story of Blood. London, Herbert Jenkins, 1958.
11. Williams, M. R., and Lindberg, D. S.: An Introduction to the Profession of Medical Technology, 3rd Ed. Philadelphia, Lea & Febiger, 1979.

Chapter 2

PROFESSIONALISM

The term professional seems to mean different things to different people. To the high school athlete, the term professional may bring to mind the name of some quarterback in the National Football League. To the stockbroker, the term is more likely to remind him of clients who are lawyers or physicians. What then characterizes a professional? In early times, those who belonged to the three learned disciplines, theology, law, or medicine, were considered professionals. As technology advanced and specialization grew, other disciplines such as education and certain levels of the business community were added to the list.

For our purposes, a professional is defined as an individual who has been extensively trained to render a particular service and is governed by an organized body that regulates continued practice in the field of training by requiring (1) adherence to a code of ethics and (2) an assessment of competency.

How many times have you heard someone say, "That person is very unprofessional!" Just what do they mean? Well, it could mean that the person was fabricating quality control results or, on the other hand, just wearing a dirty lab coat.

We have defined professional, but "acting professional" or "professionalism" is much more difficult to define, because the meaning covers such a wide range of activities. Most professional societies have a "code of ethics," a principle of right or good conduct. The code of ethics outlines what must and must not be done in order to avoid harming the life, well-being, or privacy of the recipient of that service. Laboratorians do not reveal the results of laboratory tests to anyone except authorized persons, because to do so would violate a principle of good conduct. It would be unethical, thus, unprofessional.

An example of a code of ethics is that of the American Society for Medical Technology. It is as follows:

> Being fully cognizant of my responsibilities in the practice of Medical Technology, I affirm my willingness to discharge my duties with accuracy, thoughtfulness and care.
> Realizing that the knowledge obtained concerning patients in the course of my work must be treated as confidential, I hold inviolate the confidence placed in me by patients and physicians.
> Recognizing that my integrity and that of my profession must be pledged to the absolute reliability of my work, I will conduct myself at all times in a manner appropriate to the dignity of my profession.

Like professionalism, ethics is also hard to define. Bissell and Cosman, however, put it very well when they stated that "ethics consists of far more than abiding by rules, procedures, and guidelines. . . . Ethics represents what we should do, not what we must do. It represents an expression of conscience. . . ."

In addition to honesty and confidentiality, another important aspect of professionalism is the laboratorian's personal appearance. I recall a personal experience while shopping at a hardware store. The owner of the store asked whether I was acquainted with an individual who was employed at the local hospital. I indicated that the name was familiar, but the person had resigned from the laboratory staff just before I had arrived as the laboratory director. The store owner commented, "I'm glad to hear he is no longer with you. The few times that I've had to go to the emergency room and he was on call, he came in looking like he had just finished feeding the pigs."

Appearance instills confidence. In all probability, the store owner had serious doubts about the results of the laboratory tests because he had reservations concerning the appearance of the person who came to draw his blood.

Times are changing; nevertheless, since most of the patients in general care hospitals are elderly, conservative dress is appropriate. The type of uniform to be worn is dictated by the individual hospital. Even so, it should be clean and unwrinkled. Only closed-toe, nonskid-sole shoes should be worn. They too should be as clean as possible.

Hair should be clean and long hair should be confined away from the face. The beards and mustaches of male staff members should be neatly trimmed. Otherwise, the face should be shaved, not stubbled with one- or two-days' growth.

It is a must that the hands be clean and the fingernails well groomed. Body odor should be undetectable. A fresh breath will be most appreciated, not only by patients, but by fellow employees as well. Excessive jewelry should be avoided. Only a wedding band and/or engagement or class ring should be worn on the hands. Long, dangling earrings are inappropriate (and possibly unsafe) to wear while on duty.

Although dress and grooming are extremely important aspects of professional appearance, they are not the entire picture. The laboratorian who appears unhurried, who is considerate and gentle when handling the patient, and who speaks in an authoritative but quiet voice, further enhances the patient's confidence in that laboratorian and in the results of the laboratory tests to be done.

BIBLIOGRAPHY

1. Becan-McBride, K. (ed.): Textbook of Clinical Laboratory Supervision. New York, Appleton-Century-Crofts, 1982.
2. Bissell, M., and Cosman, T.: How ethical dilemmas induce stress. Medical Laboratory Observer, *23:*28, 1991.
3. So You're Going to Collect a Blood Specimen. Skokie, IL, College of American Pathologists, 1974.
4. Williams, M. R., and Lindberg, D. S.: An Introduction to the Profession of Medical Technology, 3rd Ed. Philadelphia, Lea & Febiger, 1979.

Chapter 3

GENERAL RULES FOR SAFETY

Regulations by the Occupational Safety and Health Administration (OSHA) have caused an increased emphasis on safety in the clinical laboratory, as well as in other areas in health care settings. The Joint Commission on Accreditation of Healthcare Organizations (JCAHO), the College of American Pathologists (CAP), as well as the state governments have developed safety guidelines that must be followed for either accreditation or licensure. Unfortunately, nothing is less understood or more often ignored by laboratory personnel than safety procedures. Following is a general list of some of the safety rules that should be observed by laboratorians involved with specimen collection and preparation. The order in which they are listed has no significance. Although it would be admirable if one could remember and observe each item on this list, it is more important that each laboratory employee read and become familiar with the established Safety Procedure Manual for his own clinical laboratory. Because of the extraordinary risks associated with the hepatitis B virus and acquired immunodeficiency syndrome (AIDS), a number of the precautions listed in this chapter will be emphasized again in the chapter on infection prevention.

1. Only closed-toe, nonskid-sole shoes should be worn to work in order to prevent possible serious injuries from falls, objects accidentally dropped on the feet, or broken glassware.

2. Uniforms, or work clothes, should be neither tightly form-fitting nor floppy. Aside from looking "professional," the reasons for this are that clothes that are too tight inhibit movement and clothes that are floppy could become entangled in mechanical equipment.

3. Long hair should be secured away from the face, and beards should be neatly trimmed. Long hair (and even long beards) could become entangled in laboratory equipment. Contamination of specimens, work areas, or reagents may occur from shedding of long hair and beards.

4. Develop the habit of keeping the hands away from the mouth and eyes to prevent self-inoculation with infectious agents.

5. *Develop the habit of frequently washing the hands, particularly between patient contacts, after removal of gloves and other protective wear, before leaving the work area, before eating or drinking, after using the lavatory, and when the hands are visibly contaminated with blood, body fluids, or tissues.* For the proper handwashing procedure, refer to Chapter 4. For the recommended washing procedure for hands or skin accidentally contaminated with blood or body fluids, see Figure 4-6. *Never substitute alcohol wipes or foams when handwashing facilities are available.*

6. Never eat, smoke, or drink in the laboratory.

7. Do not store food or beverages in laboratory refrigerators used for specimen or reagent storage.

8. Always use rubber gloves to handle any specimens.

9. In preparing specimens, prevent aerosols and the resultant possible spread of infectious agents by (1) never opening the lids of centrifuges until the centrifuge has come to a complete stop and (2) only opening specimen tubes by gently twisting the stoppers and lifting them out.

10. Never pipette specimens or reagents by mouth.

11. Remove your lab coat (or other protective covering) when going to nonlaboratory areas. Change to another lab coat if it is appropriate that you wear one. When in the laboratory work area, always keep the lab coat buttoned.

12. Know the locations and types of fire extinguishers in the laboratory. Know how to use them and on what kinds of fires each type may be used.

13. Be familiar with the fire alert system, the fire escape plan, and how to report a fire in your institution.

14. Know the location and proper use of the fire blankets.

15. Know the location of all circuit breakers or master switches in the laboratory and what procedure to follow if a fellow employee should be electrocuted.

16. Know what procedure to follow if a fellow employee or patient "passes out."

17. Always make an incident report after any work-related accident, including body fluid exposure caused by injuries from sharp objects such as a needle puncture, splashes on mucous membranes, and contact with an open wound.

18. Familiarize yourself with the location and operation of all eyewash stations and safety showers.

19. Keep all reagent containers tightly closed and read all labels before using a reagent.

20. Avoid direct contact with all reagents.

21. Always properly store reagents and know the procedure for cleaning up after accidents involving reagent or body fluid spills.

22. Know where your institution keeps the Material Safety Data Sheets (MSDSs). Review their contents on a regular basis for the reagents you frequently use. This advice may appear superfluous to phlebotomists, but some of the additives in evacuated tubes are classified as hazardous chemicals.

23. Take a course in at least basic first aid and cardiopulmonary resuscitation (CPR).

24. Attend all departmental and institutional in-service programs on fire prevention and safety.

25. Know the procedure for the proper disposal of all infectious and biologic specimens, needles, and broken glassware.

26. Decontaminate bench tops after spills and at the end of each work shift.

27. Because blood-collecting trays may be a means of spreading infectious agents from one patient to another, these should be disinfected at least weekly or when visibly soiled or contaminated. Disposable trays should be replaced.

BIBLIOGRAPHY

1. Bauer, J. E.: Clinical Laboratory Methods, 9th Ed. St. Louis, C. V. Mosby, 1982.
2. Henry, J. B. (ed.): Todd-Sanford-Davidsohn Clinical Diagnosis and Management by Laboratory Methods, 17th Ed. Philadelphia, W. B. Saunders, 1984.
3. Henry, R. J., et al.: Safety in the Clinical Laboratory. Van Nuys, CA, Bio-Science Enterprises, 1976.
4. Luebbert, P. P.: Laboratory Safety and Infection Control. Chicago, ASCP Press, 1990.
5. McBride-Becan, K. (ed.): Textbook of Clinical Laboratory Supervision. New York, Appleton-Century-Crofts, 1982.
6. Centers for Disease Control: Recommendations for Prevention of HIV Transmission in Health-Care Settings. Atlanta, GA, Public Health Service, Dept. of Health and Human Services, 1987.
7. Tierno, P. M., Jr.: Preventing acquisition of human immunodeficiency virus in the laboratory: Safe handling of AIDS specimens. Lab. Med., *17:*696, 1986.

Chapter 4

INFECTION PREVENTION

Infectious disease agents are most often transmitted in one of four ways.

1. *Airborne* or *inhalation transmission,* in which a susceptible individual inhales droplets or particles of dust containing infectious agents. It is in this manner that streptococcal sore throat, respiratory viruses, and pulmonary tuberculosis can be contracted. Although coughing and sneezing most often come to mind when thinking of airborne transmissions, centrifugation and the "popping" of specimen container tops are also responsible for droplet formation.

2. *Contact transmission* can be either *direct* or *indirect.* In direct contact the causative agent is passed from one individual directly to another individual. Infections with syphilis, gonorrhea, and the human immunodeficiency virus (HIV), the virus that causes the acquired immunodeficiency syndrome (AIDS), are most commonly contracted in this manner. So too are staphylococcal infections when this bacterium is transferred from the hands of one person to the skin surface or wound of another. Hand contact, such as "shaking hands" with an infected individual, is also thought to be one of the primary ways that respiratory virus infections are spread. Individuals can be indirectly exposed to infectious agents through contact with *inanimate objects.* Examples of this include blood collection tubes, specimen containers, and pencils and pens that are contaminated on the outside with infected blood or body substances. Accidental needle sticks and the sharing of needles by drug abusers are other examples. A person can also be indirectly exposed by receiving infected blood or blood products. Hepatitis C and HIV are examples of infections spread by this route.

3. As the name implies, in *ingestion transmission* food or water containing pathogenic organisms is ingested. Contamination can result from soiled hands or insects that carry on their legs and bodies pathogenic organisms from the feces on which they feed. Salmonellosis and hepatitis A are examples of infectious agents spread in this manner. The ingestion of

pathogenic organisms can also occur via milk or eggs from infected animals. Examples include milk from cows infected with brucellosis and eggs from fowl infected with salmonella.

4. *Vectorborne transmission* occurs when an arthropod, referred to as a vector, transfers an organism. Three examples of vectorborne transmission are malaria and encephalitis, which are transmitted by mosquitoes, and Lyme disease, which is carried by ticks.

Almost 100% of the infectious agents found in the clinical laboratory are spread by either airborne (inhalation) or contact transmission. Strict adherence to universal precautions, body substance isolation, and proper handwashing will help to interrupt these chains of transmission and minimize the risk of infection.

BIOSAFETY TECHNIQUES

Universal Precautions and Body Substance Isolation

Because of the increasing prevalence of the human immunodeficiency virus (HIV), and because it is difficult to identify all patients with HIV or other bloodborne pathogens, it is prudent for phlebotomists and other laboratory personnel to take appropriate precautions for preventing the transmission of bloodborne infectious diseases. The approach of using universal precautions was recommended by the Centers for Disease Control (CDC) in 1987. The objective was to decrease the risk of exposure of healthcare workers to bloodborne diseases, such as hepatitis B and AIDS. Universal precautions, along with a further application known as Body Substance Isolation, should be consistently used for *all* patients. The following are precautions specific for those doing phlebotomy:

1. Care must be taken to avoid accidental wounds from sharp instruments contaminated with potentially infectious material. This means that needles should be neither bent after use nor reinserted into their original sheaths, but should be promptly placed in a puncture-resistant container used solely for such disposal.

2. Gloves should be worn when handling blood specimens or items that could have been contaminated with blood or other body fluids.

3. Gloves should be worn when performing phlebotomy. This is particularly important when the patient is uncooperative, when collecting capillary blood specimens, and if the phlebotomist has cuts, scratches, or other breaks in the skin.

4. Gowns should be worn while collecting a specimen if there is a possibility that clothing might be soiled with blood or other body fluids.

5. Hands should be washed thoroughly following completion of any laboratory activity, and following the removal of protective gear such as gloves, aprons, or gowns. Hands or other skin surfaces should be washed *immediately* if they become contaminated with blood (see Fig. 4-6 for recommended procedures).

6. Blood or other body fluid spills should be cleaned up promptly using

an accepted procedure. A 1:10 dilution of household bleach *prepared fresh each week* is an especially effective disinfectant.

7. Articles soiled with blood or other body fluids should be placed in special receptacles.

8. Fluid-resistant coats, aprons, or gowns should be worn while working with potentially infectious materials. These coverings should be appropriately discarded before leaving the laboratory.

9. All procedures involving, and manipulations of, potentially infectious material should be performed carefully to minimize the creation of droplets and aerosols. During procedures that are likely to generate droplets of blood or other body fluids, face protection should be worn to prevent exposure of the mucous membranes of the mouth, nose, and eyes.

10. Care should be taken when collecting specimens to avoid contaminating the outside of the container. If a specimen container is visibly contaminated with blood or other body fluids, it should be cleaned with a disinfectant. The 1:10 dilution of household bleach is appropriate for this. Specimens that are to be transported any distance should be placed in impervious bags free of leaks or cracks.

11. Evacuated specimen containers should be filled using their internal vacuum only. If a specimen is collected in a syringe and then transferred to an evacuated container, never force the fluid into the evacuated container by pressing on the syringe plunger. After puncturing the diaphragm of the evacuated container with the syringe needle, allow the correct amount of fluid to slowly flow into the evacuated container.

12. Laboratory work surfaces should be decontaminated with a disinfectant following completion of work activities.

Persons employed in health care should remember that they are bound under the legal concept of duty to care for persons who are admitted for the diagnosis and treatment of AIDS. If phlebotomists and other personnel stringently follow established standards and guidelines, all indications are that the risk of becoming infected is negligible.

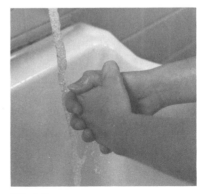

Handwashing

1. Using a mild soap, use as much friction between the two hands as possible to remove gross contamination and dead skin.

Fig. 4-1.

2. Rinse the hands well under warm running water. Hold the hands and fingers in a downward position.

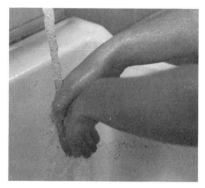

Fig. 4-2.

3. Again apply soap and vigorously wash the hands between the fingers and the wrists.

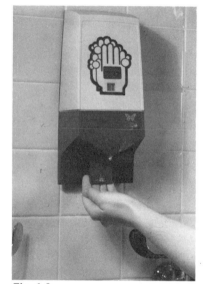

Fig. 4-3.

4. Rinse the hands in the same manner as described in paragraph number 2.

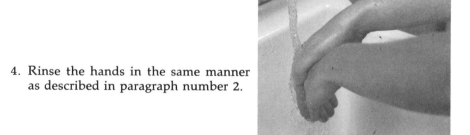

Fig. 4-4.

5. Thoroughly dry the hands, using paper towels. Turn off the water faucets, using a paper towel in order to prevent recontamination.
HANDWASHING IS THE SINGLE MOST IMPORTANT MEANS OF PREVENTING THE SPREAD OF INFECTIONS IN HOSPITALS.

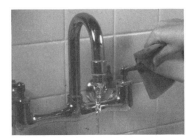

Fig. 4-5.

1. Wash with a good liquid antimicrobial detergent soap.
2. Rinse well with water.
3. Apply a solution of 50% isopropyl or ethyl alcohol.
   Leave on the skin surface for at least 1 minute.
4. Wash again with the liquid soap and rinse with water.

Fig. 4-6. Recommended washing procedure for hands or exposed skin contaminated with blood or body fluids.

Gowning, Gloving, and Masking

1. After washing your hands, put on a clean gown. The gown should be sufficiently long to cover most of your uniform, and it should have long sleeves. Pick up the gown from the inside, near the openings for the arms. Let it fall open, but do not let it touch the floor. Next, put one arm in, then the other, so that the opening is in the back. First tie the neck strings, then securely tie the waist strings.

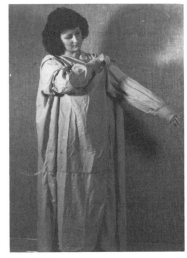

Fig. 4-7.

2. The mask should be tied high on the head so that it will not slip. Some masks have a metal band that allows one to mold the mask over the bridge of the nose for a snug fit. Masks are usually ineffective after about 20 minutes because of moisture.

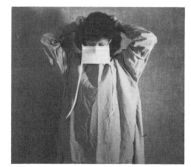

Fig. 4-8.

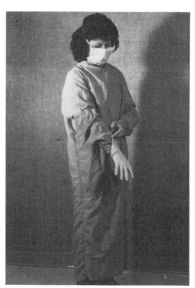

3. Next, put on the gloves and pull the ends over the sleeves of the gown (Fig. 4-9). In most cases, clean, not sterile, gloves will suffice. If sterile gloves must be used, first pick up one glove by grasping the outside of the cuff with your thumb and index finger (Fig. 4-10). Now work the glove onto the opposite hand. Next, using the index finger of the gloved hand, slip it under the cuff of the remaining glove (Fig. 4-11). Be careful not to touch the outside of the cuff. Cautiously work the other hand into the glove. Now *roll,* from the hand toward the wrist, the cuff over the sleeve of the gown. *Do not pull* the cuff over the sleeve.

Fig. 4-9.

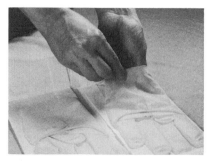

Fig. 4-10.

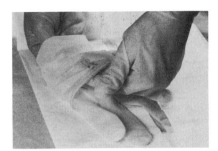

Fig. 4-11.

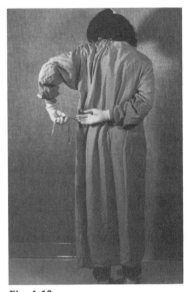

4. To remove the protective apparel, first untie the gown at the waist.

Fig. 4-12.

5. Next, remove the gloves so that you do not contaminate yourself. This is done by grasping the top edge of the gloves, which are on the sleeve of the gown, and pulling them inside out. Deposit the gloves in the proper receptacle.

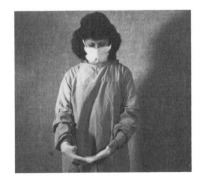

Fig. 4-13.

6. Now remove the mask by holding only the ties. Deposit it in the proper receptacle.

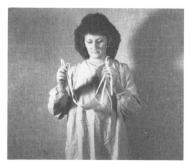

Fig. 4-14.

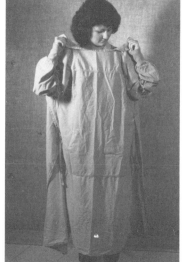

7. Untie the neck of the gown and slip it off the shoulders.

Fig. 4-15.

8. Pull the gown off so that the sleeves are inside out and the front of the gown is folded inward. Make sure the front of the gown does not come in contact with your hands or uniform.

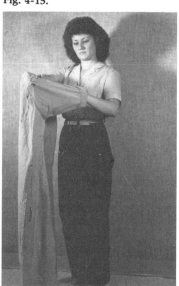

Fig. 4-16.

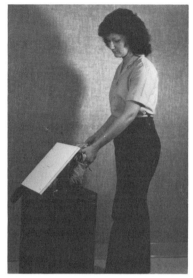

9. Deposit the gown in the proper receptacle.

Fig. 4-17.

10. Wash your hands.

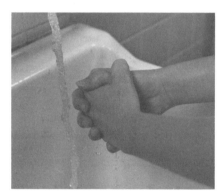

Fig. 4-18.

BIBLIOGRAPHY

1. Body Substance Isolation: Infection Control Manual. Valdosta, GA, South Georgia Medical Center, 1988.
2. Castle, M.: Hospital Infection Control, Principles and Practice. New York, John Wiley and Sons, 1980.
3. Centers for Disease Control: Recommendations for Prevention of HIV Transmission in Health-Care Settings. Atlanta, GA, Public Health Service, Dept. of Health and Human Services, 1987.
4. Leibrandt, T. (ed.): Diseases. Horsham, PA, Intermed Communications, 1981.
5. Walter, J. B.: An Introduction to the Principles of Disease. Philadelphia, W. B. Saunders, 1977.

Chapter 5

MEDICAL TERMS AND ABBREVIATIONS

Communication is an essential part of any job or profession, but nowhere is good communication more important than in health-related fields. Communication is best when one uses terms that everyone can understand. Why say that someone has "pharyngitis" when all you are trying to convey is that the person has a "sore throat"? On the other hand, sometimes general terms do not adequately describe the problem. A severe, sharp pain along the glossopharyngeal nerve causes a "sore throat." The term "glossopharyngeal neuralgia" better communicates what caused the "sore throat," and distinguishes it from other types of sore throats such as the "strep throat," which is more familiar. In other words, in medicine, as in all other professions, certain terms give exact meanings that cannot be conveyed by simpler means. It is imperative, then, that all professionals in the medical field, not just physicians and nurses, be familiar with the most frequently used medical terminology.

This section is divided into four parts. The first part gives important prefixes, suffixes, and word roots which, even if you do not know the definition of medical terms, will give you a clue to some of their meanings. The second part is a list of words or terms that should be in the vocabulary of any laboratorian. The third part is a list of often used abbreviations and symbols. The last section contains the names of commonly ordered laboratory tests and their basic clinical usefulness.

It would be negligent to end the introduction of this section without mentioning that communication is a two-way street. *Listening is just as important as talking.*

PREFIXES, SUFFIXES, AND WORD ROOTS

Word Part	Meaning	Example
a, an	without	apnea
aer/o	air	aerobic
algia	pain	neuralgia
angi/o	vessel	angiospasm
anti	against	antibiotics
arth	joint	arthritis
bi	two	bifocal
bio	life	biology
blast	embryonic cell	myeloblast
brady	slow	bradycardia
calc	stone	calcification
card	heart	cardiac
ceph	head	encephalitis
cerebr	skull	cerebrum
cut	skin	subcutaneous
cyst	bladder, hollow	cystotomy
cyte	cell	leukocyte
dent	tooth	dentist
derm	skin	epidermis
di	through	digestion
dipl	double	diplococcus
dys	difficult	dysmenorrhea
ectomy	removal	gastrectomy
emesis	vomiting	hyperemesis
emia	blood	anemia
end	within	endocardium
epi	on, upon	epidermis
erythr	red	erythrocyte
gast	stomach	gastrectomy
geri	old age	geriatrics
glyc	sweet	glycogen
gyne	woman	gynecology
hem	blood	hematology
hepat	liver	hepatic
hist	tissue	histology
hydr	water	hydrophobia
hyper	above normal	hyperthyroidism
hypo	below normal	hypoglycemia
hyster	uterus	hysterectomy
inter	between	interstitial
intra	within	intracellular
itis	inflammation	dermatitis
leuk	white	leukemia
lysis	breakdown	hemolysis
macr/o	large	macrocyte
mal	bad	malignancy

Word Part	Meaning	Example
meg	great, large	hepatomegaly
men	menses	menstruation
mening	meninges	meningitis
micr	small	microbe
morph	form	morphology
myo	muscle	myocardium
neph	kidney	nephritis
neur	nerve	neurology
noso	relating to disease	nosocomial
oma	tumor	glaucoma
onc	tumor, mass	oncolysis
orrhea	flow or discharge	pyorrhea
orth	straight, correct	orthostatic
os, oste	bone	osteomyelitis
osis	condition	sarcoidosis
otomy	incision	duodenotomy
par	to give birth to	postpartum
para	beside, near	parathyroid
path	sick	pathogenic
penia	decrease in	leukopenia
peri	around	pericardium
phleb	vein	phlebotomy
pneum	air	pneumonia
poly	many	polycythemia
post	behind (position)	postnasal
post	after (time)	postpartum
pre	in front of (position)	prehyoid
pre	before (time)	prenatal
psych	mind	psychosis
pulm	lung	pulm
py, pyr	fever, heat	pyrexia
pyel	renal	pyelonephritis
rhin	nose	rhinorrhea
salping	fallopian tube	salpingitis
sanguin	bloody	sanguinal
scler	hard	sclerotic
stasis	act or condition of stopping	hemostasis
sub	below, under	subacute
tach	rapid	tachycardia
thromb	clot	thrombosis
tox	poison	antitoxin
tri	three	tricuspid
ven	vein	venesection

WORDS AND TERMS

Word/Term	Meaning
Accessioning	the first step in processing a specimen, when you give it a specific number or code

Word/Term	Meaning
Accuracy	as near to the real answer as possible
Acrocyanosis	a blueness of the hands or feet caused by disturbances to the superficial veins
Adenoma	a tumor of glandular superficial epithelium
Aerobic	lives in the presence of oxygen
Allergy	an abnormal (hypersensitive) reaction to an agent or condition
Anaerobic	able to live without oxygen
Anastomosis	a communication between two vessels, either end to end or by means of a connecting channel
Anemia	deficiency of red blood cells, hemoglobin, or both
Aneurysm	a bulge in an artery caused by a weakening of its wall
Anorexia	loss of appetite
Antibiotic	a substance used in the treatment of infectious diseases, usually caused by bacteria
Antibody	A protective body protein produced as a result of exposure to an antigen
Anticoagulant	a substance that delays or prevents the blood from clotting
Antigen	a substance that stimulates a specific resistance response and thus causes the body to produce antibodies
Antimicrobial	a substance that either kills or inhibits microscopic organisms
Apnea	a temporary cessation of breathing
Arteriosclerosis	hardening of the arteries
Asepsis	free from germs or infection
Bacteria	one-cell microscopic organisms that either cause disease (pathogenic) or do not cause disease (nonpathogenic); many different kinds of bacteria normally live on the skin and in the intestine, and are referred to as "normal flora"
Bacteriology	the study of bacteria
Bacteriostatic	inhibits, but does not kill bacteria
Bradycardia	slow heartbeat
Carcinogenic	anything that is capable of or conducive to the production of cancer
Carcinoma	a malignant tumor (cancer)
Cardiology	that branch of medicine that deals with heart disease
Cardiovascular	pertaining to the heart and blood vessels
Carrier	a person who is able to spread to others a disease with which he is infected, but of which he usually has no symptoms
Centrifuge	a piece of laboratory equipment that spins test tubes at high speed and separates the cellular and liquid portions of the blood
Cephalgia	headache

Word/Term	Meaning
Clot	coagulated blood
Coagulate	to change from a fluid state into a semisolid mass
Coccus	a type of bacterium that is spherical in form
Collateral	side by side, subordinate
Communicable	refers to a communicable disease that may be spread from one person to another either directly or indirectly
Coumadin	an anticoagulant or blood-thinning agent also known as warfarin; prothrombin time determinations are essential for its proper control
Crenated	notched red blood cells
Croup	a childhood disease that is characterized by a barking cough and difficult breathing
Cyanosis	a condition in which the skin turns a bluish color because of lack of oxygen to the blood
Cystic fibrosis	an inherited disorder of the exocrine glands that causes them to produce thick secretions of mucus; obstruction of the small bowel and persistent upper respiratory infections may result
Cystitis	inflammation of the urinary bladder
Differential	a percentage of each type of white blood cell in a total of 100 white cells observed
Digoxin	a drug used to strengthen heart contractions, also known as Lanoxin
Disinfect	to kill disease-causing germs
Dysentery	a diarrhea in which blood or mucus or both may be present in the feces
Dyspnea	difficulty in breathing
Ectopic	away from or out of the normal location
Edema	a condition in which the body tissues contain an excessive amount of fluid, resulting in swelling
Embolus	a blood clot or some other mass (which may be solid, liquid, or gaseous) that stops up a blood vessel, brought to the plugged vessel from another area
Emphysema	a chronic disease of the lungs in which there is an improper exchange of oxygen and carbon dioxide
Empyema	pus in a body cavity, especially in the chest cavity
Encephalitis	inflammation of the brain
Endocarditis	inflammation of the inner lining of the heart, including the heart valves
Endocrine	pertains to a group of ductless glands that secrete a substance or hormone that affects other organs directly into the bloodstream
Endocrinology	that branch of medicine that deals with diseases of the ductless glands, e.g., pituitary or thyroid glands
Endogenous	Something produced within a cell or organism

Word/Term	Meaning
Endothelium	a layer of flat cells that lines the inner surface of the entire circulatory system
Enteric	pertaining to the intestinal tract
Enzyme	a complex compound that is able to initiate chemical changes in the body
Epithelium	a layer of cells that covers the internal and external surfaces of the body
Exocrine	secretion through a narrow tubular structure (duct) that opens onto an organ, tissue, or vessel
Exogenous	something produced outside a cell or organism—for example, endogenous obesity would be caused by a dysfunction of the metabolic systems, whereas exogenous obesity would be caused by eating too many high-calorie foods
Exudate	fluid secreted by tissue, which may occur normally, but is usually in response to inflammation, damage, or irritation
Febrile	with fever
Fibrillation	quivering of the heart muscle rather than normal contraction
Fistula	an abnormal, tubelike canal extending from one organ to another
Gastralgia	stomachache
Gastritis	inflammation of the lining of the stomach
Gastroenterology	that branch of medicine concerned with the physiology and pathology of the stomach, intestines, and related areas
Gastrointestinal	having to do with the stomach and intestines
Gauge	as used in the laboratory, a unit of measurement determining the dimension of a needle
Geriatric	that branch of medicine that deals with the health and diseases of the elderly
Germicide	a substance that kills germs
Glomerulonephritis	inflammation of the filtering units of the kidneys
Gram stain	a special stain used to help classify bacteria into two groups: gram-positive and gram-negative
Gynecology	that branch of medicine that deals with diseases of the female reproductive organs
Hematocrit	a laboratory test in which the red blood cells are centrifuged at a high speed so they will be separated from the blood serum and their volume can be expressed as a percentage of the total volume
Hematology	the study of blood and its diseases
Hematoma	a mass of blood that is collected in the tissue and is caused by a break in a blood vessel
Hemoconcentration	a rapid increase in the relative red blood cell content in the blood
Hemolysis	destruction of the red blood cells

Word/Term	Meaning
Hemophilia	a hereditary disease characterized by a prolonged clotting time of the blood
Hemorrhage	abnormal internal or external bleeding
Hepatic	having to do with the liver
Hepatitis	inflammation of the liver usually resulting from an infection by a transmissible virus
Hepatomegaly	enlarged liver
Hormone	a substance that is produced by a ductless gland and is carried to other parts of the body by the blood; it exerts control over many of the body's processes
Host	a plant or animal in which a parasite lives
Hyperglycemia	excessive amount of sugar in the blood
Hyperkalemia	an excess of potassium in the blood
Hyperlipidemia	a general term meaning an excess of any or all kinds of lipids in the plasma
Hypernatremia	an excess of sodium in the blood
Hypochromic	a decrease of iron pigment in the red blood cells
Hypoglycemia	a condition in which the blood sugar level is too low
Hypokalemia	a decrease of potassium in the blood
Hyponatremia	a decrease of sodium in the blood
Hysterectomy	surgical removal of the uterus
Ileitis	inflammation of the ileum, which is the terminal portion of the small intestine
Immune	a condition in which the body is able to resist certain illnesses or toxins
Incubation	maintenance at a specified temperature and for a specified time until growth or a reaction occurs
Infarct	death of a segment of tissue, resulting from a lack of blood supply to that area
Infection	invasion of the body by bacteria, molds, viruses, or parasites
Inoculate	to put into the body a substance (vaccine) that will cause the body to produce antibodies
Insulin	a natural hormone that is produced by the pancreas and is involved with the metabolism of blood sugar; diabetic individuals are not able to secrete proper amounts of their own insulin
Intercellular	located between the cells
Interstitial	pertains to that which occupies the space between the tissues
Ischemia	a temporary deficiency of blood to a localized area, caused by an obstruction
Isolation	the limitation of movement and social contact of a patient

Word/Term	Meaning
Ketosis	an accumulation in the body of substances known as ketones, which may be detected by testing urine; it is commonly observed in starvation, pregnancy, and diabetes
Laryngitis	inflammation of the larynx
Leukemia	a blood disease in which there is an overproduction of white blood cells
Leukocytes	a broad term covering all types of white blood cells
Leukocytosis	an increase in the number of white blood cells
Leukopenia	a decrease in the number of white blood cells
Lipemic	the presence of an abnormal amount of fatty substance
Liter	a metric fluid measure of 1000 milliliters; approximately 2 pints
Lithium	a psychoactive agent used in the treatment of manic-depressive disorders
Lysis	the dissolution of a red blood cell
Mastitis	inflammation of the breast
Megalocardia	enlarged heart
Melanoma	a malignant tumor that is often black
Menorrhagia	excessive menstrual flow
Metacarpal	having to do with the hands
Metatarsal	having to do with the feet
Microbiology	the study of microscopic organisms
Milliliter	1/1000 of a liter
Monilia	an outdated term indicating an infection with the yeast *Candida albicans;* candidiasis is the proper term
Morphology	the study of structure
Multiple myeloma	a disease characterized by the formation of multiple tumor masses in the bone and bone marrow
Multiple sclerosis	a chronic, slowly progressive disease of the nervous system
Myocarditis	inflammation of the heart muscle
Myxedema	a condition caused by the underfunctioning of the thyroid gland
Neonatal	the first 6 weeks after birth
Neoplasm	new growth, such as a tumor
Nephritis	inflammation of the kidney
Nephrology	the science of the function and structure of the kidneys
Neurology	that branch of medicine that deals with the nervous system and its diseases
Nosocomial	pertaining to a hospital; a nosocomial infection would be one obtained while in a hospital
Obstetrics	that branch of medicine concerned with women during pregnancy and childbirth
Oncology	that branch of medicine that deals with tumors

Word/Term	Meaning
Ophthalmology	that branch of medicine that deals with the eye and its diseases
Orthopedic	that branch of medicine that deals with problems of the skeleton, joints, muscles, and other supporting structures
Otitis	inflammation of the ear; the area is differentiated, e.g., otitis media means inflammation of the middle ear
Otorrhea	a discharge from the ear
Palpate	to examine by touching with the fingers
Palpitation	a rapid, intense beating of the heart
Pancreatitis	inflammation of the pancreas
Patent	open where fluid such as blood can flow freely; we say that a vein is patent if the vein still has its elasticity or if there is no blockage because of scar tissue
Pathogenic	anything that can produce a disease
Pathology	the study of structural or functional changes in body tissues and organs caused by a disease
Pediatrics	that branch of medicine related to the care and treatment of diseases of children
Pharyngitis	inflammation of the pharynx
Phlebitis	the inflammation of a vein, often accompanied by clot formation
Prandial	pertains to a meal and is used in relation to timing, as in "2-hour postprandial" or 2 hours after a meal
Precision	to repeat a procedure several times and be able to obtain nearly the same answer every time
Proctology	that branch of medicine that deals with the diagnosis and treatment of diseases of the anus, rectum, and colon
Psychiatry	that branch of medicine that deals with mental illness
Pulmonary	refers to the lungs and lung tissue
Renal	relating to the kidney
Respiratory	having to do with respiration or, more specifically, the taking in of oxygen and the release of carbon dioxide by the lungs
Rod	a nonspecific name for a group of bacteria that generally have the shape of a slender, straight bar
Salpingitis	inflammation of the fallopian tubes
Sclerosis	a general term indicating the abnormal hardening of tissue
Sepsis	an infection of the blood with a pathogenic organism or a product (toxin) produced by the organism
Serology	the testing of blood serum for antigen-antibody reactions
Shunt	to divert flow from one main route to another

Word/Term	Meaning
Sterile	the absence of living microorganisms
Susceptible	a condition in which a person is more than normally vulnerable to a disease
Syncope	a fainting spell
Thrombophlebitis	inflammation of the wall of a vein with an accompanying clot at the site
Thrombosis	the formation of a blood clot called a thrombus, which remains at the site of its formation in the circulatory system; when it becomes detached, it is known as an embolus
Transmission	the spreading of a disease from one person to another
Transudate	a fluid that has diffused through the capillaries; it differs from an exudate in that it has fewer cellular elements
Urinary	having to do with the urinary tract or urine
Urology	that branch of medicine concerned with the urinary tract of both sexes and the genital tract of males
Vaginitis	inflammation of the vagina
Vascular	refers to the blood system; also describes tissue heavily supplied with blood vessels
Vasoconstrictor	an agent that causes a decrease in the diameter of a blood vessel; this condition may be caused by either the introduction of a drug or a disease condition
Vasodilator	refers to an agent that causes an increase in the diameter of a blood vessel, thus producing greater blood flow
Virology	the study of viruses, infectious agents that are too small to be seen through the usual light microscope

GENERAL ABBREVIATIONS

Abbreviations	Meaning
a.c.	before meals (*ante cibum*)
ad lib	as desired (*ad libitum*)
AIDS	acquired immunodeficiency syndrome
ASAP	as soon as possible
ASCP	American Society of Clinical Pathologists
b.i.d.	twice a day (*bis in die*)
B/P	blood pressure
Ca	cancer
CLS	clinical laboratory scientist
CLT	clinical laboratory technician
cm	centimeter
COPD	chronic obstructive pulmonary disease
CPR	cardiopulmonary resuscitation

Abbreviations	Meaning
CPT	certified phlebotomy technician
CVA	cardiovascular/cerebrovascular accident
D & C	dilation and curettage
DOA	dead on arrival
DOB	date of birth
ECG	electrocardiogram
EEG	electroencephalogram
EKG	electrocardiogram (ECG is preferred abbreviation)
ENT	eyes, nose, and throat
E.R.	emergency room
FUO	fever of unknown origin
GI	gastrointestinal
gtt	drops (guttac)
HCFA	Health Care Financing Administration
h.s.	hours of sleep
IM	intramuscular
I & O	intake and output
IV	intravenous
LP	lumbar puncture
L.P.N.	licensed practical nurse
MI	myocardial infarction
MLT	medical laboratory technician
MT	medical technologist
NPO	nothing by mouth (*non per os*)
OD	overdose
O.R.	operating room
p.c.	after food (*post cibum*)
PDR	Physician's Desk Reference
PP	postprandial (after a meal)
p.r.n.	whenever necessary (*pro re nata*)
q.d.	every day (*quaque die*)
q.h.	every hour
q2h	every 2 hours
q.i.d.	four times a day (*quater in die*)
QNS	quantity not sufficient
q.o.d.	every other day
q.s.	as much as will suffice (*quantum sufficit*)
R.N.	registered nurse
SBE	subacute bacterial endocarditis
SOB	short of breath
stat	to be done immediately (*statim*)
t.i.d.	three times a day (*ter in die*)
TPR	temperature/pulse/respiration
TUR	transurethral resection
URI	upper respiratory infection
UTI	urinary tract infection

OFTEN USED CLINICAL LABORATORY ABBREVIATIONS

Abbreviations	Meaning
Ab	antibody
ABO	blood types
AFB	acid-fast bacillus
AFP	alphafetoprotein
ALT	alanine aminotransferase (SGPT)
ANA	antinuclear antibody
anti-HBc	hepatitis B core antibody
anti-HBe	hepatitis B e antibody
anti-HBs	hepatitis B surface antibody
APTT	activated partial thromboplastin time (PTT)
ASO	antistreptolysin-O
AST	aspartate aminotransferase (SGOT)
BT	bleeding time
BUN	blood urea nitrogen
Ca	calcium
CBC	complete blood count
CEA	carcinoembryonic antigen
CMV	cytomegalovirus
CPK/CK	creatinine phosphokinase
CRP	C-reactive protein
CSF	cerebrospinal fluid
C3/C4	complement
C50/C100	total complement
DIC	disseminated intravascular coagulation
diff	white blood cell differential
EBV	Epstein-Barr virus
ESR	erythocyte sedimentation rate
FBS	fasting blood sugar
FDP	fibrin degradation product
FSH	follicle-stimulating hormone
FTA	fluorescent treponemal antibody
GC	gonorrhea
g/dl	grams per deciliter
GTT	glucose tolerance test
HAA	hepatitis-associated antigen (HBsAg)
HAV	hepatitis A virus
HBcAb	hepatitis B core antibody (anti-HBc)
HBeAb	hepatitis B e antibody (anti-HBe)
HBeAg	hepatitis B e antigen
HBsAb	hepatitis B surface antibody (anti-HBs)
HBsAg	hepatitis B surface antigen (HAA)
hCG	human chronionic gonadotropin
HCl	hydrochloric acid
Hct	hematocrit
HCV	heptitis C virus (non-A, non-B hepatitis)
HDL	high-density lipoprotein (cholesterol)
HDV	hepatitis D (delta) virus
Hgb	hemaglobin

Abbreviations	Meaning
HIV	human immunodeficiency virus (the AIDS virus)
HLA	human leukocyte antigens
HPF	high-power field
HPL	human placental lactogen
HSV	herpes simplex virus
HTLV-I	human T-lymphocyte virus I (the virus that causes T-cell acute lymphocyte leukemia)
HTLV-III	human T-lymphocyte virus III (the old designation for the AIDS virus; see HIV)
IU	international unit
K	potassium
Kg	kilogram
KOH	potassium hydroxide
LD/LDH	lactate dehydrogenase
LDL	low density lipoprotein (cholesterol)
LE	lupus erythematosus
Li	lithium
LPF	low-power field
MCH	mean corpuscular hemoglobin
MCHC	mean cell hemoglobin concentration
MCV	mean corpuscular volume
mEq/L	milliequivalent per liter
mg	milligram
ml/mL	milliliter
mm	millimeter
mm^3	cubic millimeter
Na	sodium
NaOH	sodium hydroxide
O & P	ova and parasites
PAP	prostate acid phosphatase
Pap	Papanicolaou's stain
PKU	phenylketonuria
PSA	prostate-specific antigen
PT	prothrombin time
PTT	partial thromboplastin time (APTT)
RBC	red blood count/red blood cells
retic	reticulocyte
Rh	blood factor (Rhesus) reported as negative or positive, usually with the blood type (e.g., O positive)
RMSF	Rocky Mountain spotted fever
RPR	rapid plasma reagin; test for syphilis
RSV	respiratory syncytial virus
sed rate	sedimentation rate
SGOT	serum glutamicoxaloacetic transaminase (AST)
SGPT	serum glutamicpyruvic transaminase (ALT)
SLE	systemic lupus erythematosus
SMA	sequential multiple analyzer/smooth muscle antibody
STD	sexually transmitted disease
STS	serologic test for syphillis

Abbreviations	Meaning
TB	tuberculosis
TIBC	total iron binding capacity
TP	total protein
TSH	thyroid-stimulating hormone
UA	urinalysis/uric acid
VDRL	Veneral Disease Research Laboratory; test for syphilis
VLDL	very low density lipoprotein (cholesterol)
WBC	white blood count/white blood cell
X-match	cross match of blood for transfusion

SYMBOLS

Symbol	Meaning
$\bar{c}$	with
P_{CO_2}	blood gas symbol—partial pressure of carbon dioxide
P_{O_2}	blood gas symbol—partial pressure of oxygen
$\bar{s}$	without
μ	micron
↑	elevated
↓	decreased
>	greater than
<	less than
≥	equal to or greater than
≤	equal to or less than
≅	approximately equal to
R_x	prescription
1+	slight trace
2+	trace
3+	moderate
4+	large amount

COMMONLY ORDERED LABORATORY TESTS

Test	Basic Clinical Usefulness
Acid phosphatase	prostatic cancer
Alanine aminotransferase (ALT/ SGPT)	hepatic disease
Alkaline phosphatase	skeletal disease and hepatic disorders
Alphafetoprotein (AFP)	assist in the diagnosis of hepatic disorders and some neural tube congenital defects
Ammonia	severe hepatic disease
Amylase	pancreatitis
Antinuclear antibody (ANA)	screen for autoimmune disease, SLE, and chronic active hepatitis
Antistreptolysin O titer (ASO)	document exposure to streptococcal infection

Test	Basic Clinical Usefulness
Aspartate aminotransferase (AST/SGOT)	acute hepatic disease, recent myocardial infarction
Bilirubin	evaluate liver function and aid in the diagnosis of hemolytic anemia and biliary obstruction
Bleeding time	assess hemostatic function
Blood culture	diagnosis of bacteremia
Blood urea nitrogen (BUN)	evaluate renal function
Calcium	neuromuscular, skeletal, and endocrine disorders; blood-clotting deficiencies and acid-base imbalance
Cardiac isoenzymes	rule out coronary heart disease
Cholesterol	assess risk of coronary heart disease
Chorionic gonadotropin (hCG)	pregnancy
Complete blood count (CBC)	includes red and white blood count, hemoglobin, hematocrit, and differential
Coombs'	the direct Coombs' detects proteins (antibodies) that coat the red blood cell; the indirect Coombs' detects for antibodies in serum
Creatinine	assess glomerular filtration
Creatinine phosphokinase (CK/CPK)	diagnose acute MI
C-reactive protein	indicator of inflammation
Electrolytes (sodium, potassium, chloride, carbon dioxide)	acid-base balance
Ferritin	assist in diagnosis of certain anemias and evaluate total body storage of iron
Fibrin degradation products (FDP)	helpful in diagnosis of DIC
Folic acid	evaluate certain anemias and detect deficiency because folic acid is important in metabolic energy–related processes
Gamma glutamyl transferase (GGT)	useful in diagnosis of obstructive jaundice, carcinoma of pancreas and liver, and chronic alcoholic liver disease
Glucose (blood sugar) (FBS)	screen for diabetes mellitus
Glucose tolerance test (GTT)	confirm diabetes mellitus or hypoglycemia
Hematocrit	aid in diagnosis of anemia
Hemoglobin	measure severity of anemia
Iron	differential diagnosis of certain anemias
Lactic dehydrogenase (LD/LDH)	differential diagnosis of myocardial or pulmonary infarction, anemia, or hepatic disease

Test	Basic Clinical Usefulness
Lipase	diagnosis of pancreatitis
Lipid profile	evaluation of hyperlipidemia
Osmolality, serum	evaluation of electrolytes, water balance, hydration states, and liver disease
Partial thromboplastin time (PTT/ APTT)	screen for deficiencies of clotting factors
Phenylketonuria (PKU)	screening for PKU in newborns and prevention of mental retardation
Phosphorus	evaluation of alcoholism and of parathyroid and kidney disease
Platelet count	evaluation of platelet production
Prostate-specific antigen (PSA)	levels correlate with extent of prostate cancer
Protein	hepatic disease, protein deficiency, renal disorders
Prothrombin time (PT)	evaluate extrinsic coagulation
Rapid plasma reagin (RPR)	assist in diagnosis of syphilis
Red blood count (RBC)	support other tests in the diagnosis of anemia
Reticulocyte count	evaluate red blood cell production
Sickle cell preparation	detection of sickle cell disease
Thyroid-stimulating hormone (TSH)	evaluation of thyroid function
Total iron binding capacity (TIBC)	differential diagnosis of certain anemias
Triglycerides	hyperlipidemia
Uric acid	gout, kidney dysfunction
White cell count (WBC)	detect inflammation or infection

BIBLIOGRAPHY

1. Dacunha, J. P., Ford, R. D., and Glover, S. M. (eds.): Diagnostics. Springfield, IL, Intermed Communications, 1981.
2. Garb, S.: Laboratory Tests in Common Use, 6th Ed. New York, Springer, 1976.
3. Hamilton, H. D. (ed.): Definitions. Springhouse, PA, Intermed Communications, 1983.
4. Handbook of Current Medical Abbreviations. Bowie, MD, The Charles Press, 1976.
5. Henry, J. B. (ed.): Todd-Sanford-Davidsohn Clinical Diagnosis and Management by Laboratory Methods, 17th Ed. Philadelphia, W. B. Saunders, 1984.
6. Jacobs, D. S., Kasten, B. L., Jr., DeMott, W. R., and Wolfson, W. L. (eds.): Laboratory Test Handbook, 2nd Ed. Baltimore, Williams & Wilkins, 1990.
7. Kaplan, A., and Szabo, L. L.: Clinical Chemistry: Interpretation and Techniques, 3rd Ed. Philadelphia, Lea & Febiger, 1988.
8. Smith, G. L., and Davis, P. E.: Medical Terminology, 4th Ed. New York, John Wiley and Sons, 1981.
9. Stedman's Medical Dictionary, 25th Ed. Baltimore, Williams & Wilkins, 1990.
10. Stegeman, W.: Medical Terms Simplified. St. Paul, Minnesota, West Publ., 1976.
11. Tietz, N. W. (ed.): Fundamentals of Clinical Chemistry, 2nd Ed. Philadelphia, W. B. Saunders, 1976.

Chapter 6

HOW THE HEART AND CIRCULATION WORK

THE COMPOSITION OF BLOOD

If a tube of blood is allowed to stand undisturbed, it will separate into two major components. One component is red and contains the cellular portion of the blood. The other component is yellowish and can be either clear or hazy in composition. This is the liquid portion of the blood. The liquid portion is called either *plasma* or *serum,* depending on whether anticoagulants have been added to the blood sample (see Figures 6-1 and 6-2).

Anticoagulants, as the name implies, prevent the blood from coagulating or forming a clot. (Anticoagulants and coagulation will be discussed in later sections.) The blood contains a protein substance called *fibrinogen.* Under proper conditions, this substance is converted into another substance called *fibrin.* The fibrin forms a network that traps the cellular portion of the blood. This is known as the *clot.* The remaining liquid portion is known as *serum.* Because the fibrinogen was converted into fibrin to form to clot, *serum contains no fibrinogen.*

If an anticoagulant is added to the blood, it will not allow the fibrinogen to be converted into fibrin. No clot will form. Now when the blood sample separates into the two components, the liquid portion is known as *plasma. Plasma contains fibrinogen.*

The function of the red blood cells and plasma is to carry oxygen and nourishment to all parts of the body and, at the same time, to pick up waste products from the tissues to be excreted by the kidneys and lungs.

The adult body contains around 5 to 6 liters or approximately 1½ gallons of blood. Of this 1½ gallons, about 55% is composed of the liquid or fluid portion. The cellular portion of the blood makes up the remaining 45%.

The cellular portion is composed of red blood cells (erythrocytes), white blood cells (leukocytes), and platelets (thrombocytes).

In general, the red blood cell is simply a solution of hemoglobin that is contained within a membrane. Its life span is between 100 and 120 days. In

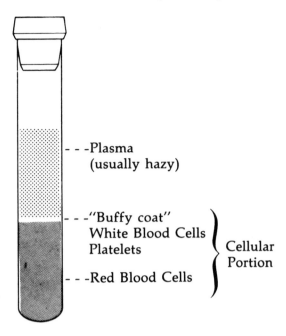

- - -Plasma
(usually hazy)

- - -"Buffy coat"
White Blood Cells
Platelets

} Cellular
Portion

- - -Red Blood Cells

Fig. 6-1. Anticoagulated blood sample.

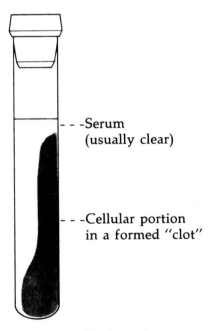

- - -Serum
(usually clear)

- - -Cellular portion
in a formed "clot"

Fig. 6-2. Nonanticoagulated blood sample.

the adult, red cells are produced in the bone marrow of the axial skeleton and proximal ends of the long bone (see Figure 6-3). The normal red cell is a biconcave disc (see Figure 6-4), which has an average diameter of 7.5 to 8.3 microns (approximately 7/25,000 of an inch).

The white blood cells are produced by the lymph nodes, spleen, thymus, and bone marrow. There are five main types of white blood cells: the neutrophilic series, eosinophilic series, basophilic series, lymphocytic series, and the monocytic series. Examples of the normal mature forms of each series are illustrated in Figure 6-5.

The entire series of white blood cells is designed to defend the body against foreign substances; however, each of the types of cells, neutrophils, monocytes, and the others, has a different function. One of the main differences between red cells and white cells is that the red cells function intravascularly (within the veins and capillaries), whereas the white cells function extravascularly (in the tissues, outside the veins and capillaries). They simply use the veins and capillaries (the blood) as roads to get from one place to another.

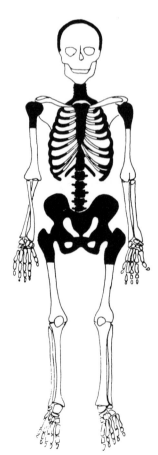

Fig. 6-3. Red cell marrow distribution in the adult.

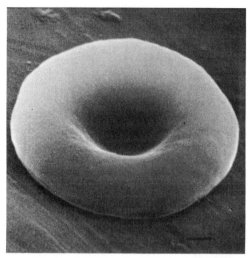

Fig. 6-4. The normal mature erythrocyte as visualized by the scanning electron microscope (×9800). (Courtesy of Dr. Wallace N. Jensen.) (From Wintrobe, M. M., et al.: Clinical Hematology, 8th Ed. Philadelphia, Lea & Febiger, 1981.)

The remaining cellular elements in the blood are the platelets. Platelets function primarily in the stoppage of bleeding. They are produced directly from the cytoplasm of a large cell called the megakaryocyte and have a life span of 9 to 12 days.

THE HEART

The heart is a highly muscular organ, containing four chambers. The two upper chambers are called the *atria;* the two lower chambers are called *ventricles.* The heart is surrounded by a fibrous sac called the *pericardium.* This sac helps to hold the heart in position and isolates it from the other contents of the chest (thoracic cavity). The inner surfaces and cavities of the heart are lined with a thin but very strong membrane called the *endocardium.* If the pericardium becomes inflamed, the condition is called *pericarditis.* Inflammation of the endocardium is referred to as *endocarditis.*

The following outline explains the circulation of the blood through the heart in more detail. Unless instructed otherwise, the reader should refer to the diagram showing the exploded view of the heart (Fig. 6-6).

1. Returning blood enters the *right atrium* from the *inferior* and *superior vena cava.*

2. The blood then flows from the right atrium through the *tricuspid valve,* filling the *right ventricle.* The tricuspid valve is one of four valves located in the heart. These valves control the direction and flow of blood through the heart.

3. As the right ventricle fills with blood, an electrical impulse is delivered, causing the right atrium to contract, thus completing the filling of the right ventricle.

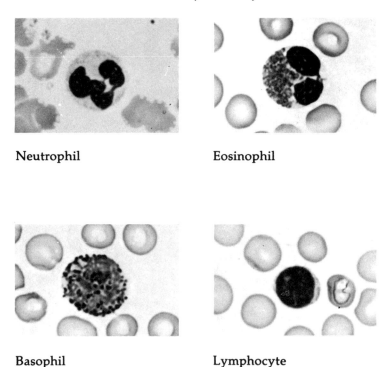

Neutrophil   Eosinophil

Basophil   Lymphocyte

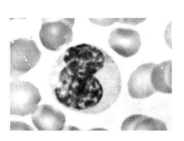

Monocyte

Fig. 6-5. Photographs of mature white blood cells. (From Brown, B. A.: Hematology: Principles and Procedures, 4th Ed. Philadelphia, Lea & Febiger, 1984.)

4. The heart has the unique ability to initiate its own electrical impulses without any stimulation from the brain. (Refer to Figure 6-7, the conduction system of the heart.) The conduction system of the heart is composed of four structures: the *sinoatrial node* or SA node (also known as the pacemaker), the *atrioventricular node* or AV node, the *AV bundle* or bundle of His, and *Purkinje fibers*. These structures are modified cardiac muscle, which differ in function from ordinary cardiac muscle. The initial impulse takes

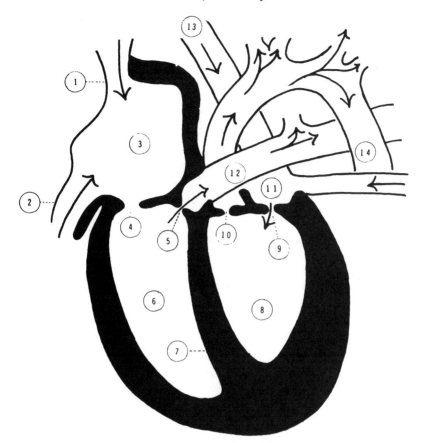

Fig. 6-6. Exploded view of the heart.

1. Superior Vena Cava
2. Inferior Vena Cava
3. Right Atrium
4. Tricuspid Valve
5. Pulmonary Valve
6. Right Ventricle
7. Septum
8. Left Ventricle
9. Mitral (Bicuspid) Valve
10. Aortic Valve
11. Left Atrium
12. Pulmonary Artery
13. Pulmonary Vein
14. Aorta

place at the SA node, which is located at the junction of the right atrium and the superior vena cava. The impulse travels first through the atria, causing them to contract. As the impulse reaches the AV node (located in the right atrium near the septum), it slows down a bit so that the atria can completely contract before the ventricles are stimulated. After the electrical impulse passes through the AV node, it picks up velocity as it is relayed through the AV bundle into the ventricles by the Purkinje fibers. This causes the ventricles to contract almost simultaneously. These electrical impulses are delivered at precisely timed intervals.

5. In reality, the heart is a double pump. Both sides perform almost simultaneously, sending blood to different places. In other words, when the right atrium contracts, the left atrium contracts at about the same time. The same is true for the right and left ventricles. (See the cardiac cycle, Figure 6-8.)

6. When the right ventricle is full, it is stimulated by the electrical impulse to begin contraction. As the pressure within the ventricle increases, it causes the tricuspid valve to close. This prevents the blood from flowing backwards into the right atrium.

7. As the ventricular pressure continues to increase, it not only causes the tricuspid valve to close, but forces the blood through the *pulmonary valve* into the *pulmonary artery,* where it flows to the lungs.

8. At the end of the ventricular contraction, the pulmonary valve closes, so that the blood, just expelled, will not flow back into the ventricles.

9. The oxygen-rich blood now returns to the heart via the *pulmonary veins.* These veins empty the blood into the *left atrium.*

10. The blood flows from the left atrium, through the *mitral valve,* filling the *left ventricle.*

11. An electrical impulse is delivered from the SA node.

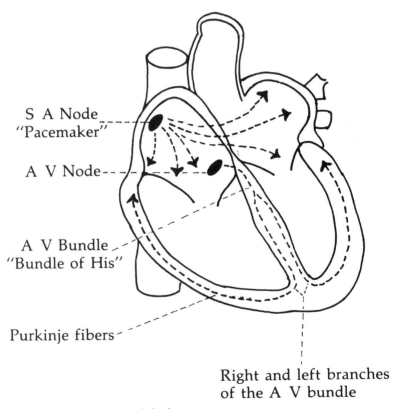

Fig. 6-7. The conduction system of the heart.

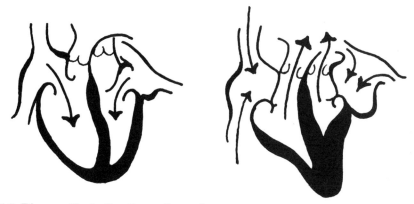

Fig. 6-8. Diagram illustrating the cardiac cycle. Note that the blood flows from both atria simultaneously and that both ventricles contract at approximately the same time.

12. The left atrium contracts, thus completing the filling of the left ventricle.

13. When the left ventricle is filled, the electrical impulse stimulates the ventricle to begin contraction. As the pressure within the ventricle increases, it causes the mitral valve to close, thus preventing a backward flow of blood into the left atrium.

14. At the same time, this ventricular pressure forces the blood through the *aortic valve* into the *aorta* to circulate throughout the body.

15. At the end of the contraction, the aortic valve closes to prevent the backflow of blood.

The heart is composed of a specialized muscle called *cardiac muscle.* The muscular wall of the heart is referred to as the *myocardium.* Like other muscles, it contracts and relaxes (approximately 72 times per minute); but unlike other muscles, it never completely rests.

The average weight of the heart is between 250 to 300 grams, and its size is approximately that of an adult fist. Like all other organs in the body, the heart must also have an adequate supply of blood to function properly. Although its chambers are continually filled with blood, the heart cannot directly use this for its own needs. So just like other organs of the body, it receives its blood from the aorta. The first two branches of the aorta, the left and right coronary arteries, supply the heart with its blood needs. If, for some reason, the smaller arteries branching from the *left* and *right coronary arteries* become closed (occluded) so that blood cannot pass through, necrosis of the cardiac muscle will occur. This is called a *myocardial infarction* or, more commonly, a "heart attack."

VEINS AND ARTERIES

Anatomy

Veins and arteries have walls constructed of three coats (see Figure 6-9). The inner coat, also called the *tunica interna* or *intima,* is composed of (1) simple

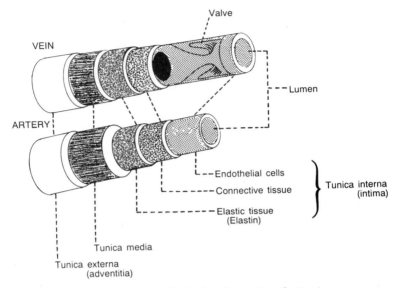

Fig. 6-9. Comparative structures of a vein (top) and an artery (bottom).

squamous epithelial cells, which line the lumen of the vessel, (2) a connective tissue layer, and (3) a layer of elastic fibers called *elastin*. The middle coat, or *tunica media,* is composed primarily of smooth muscle. The *tunica externa* or *adventitia* is the outermost layer or coat. It is composed principally of connective tissue. Although both veins and arteries have the same basic structure, arteries have relatively more muscle for their size than do veins. Because of this, arteries appear rounder than veins.

The blood pressure in the veins is insufficient to return blood to the heart, particularly from areas like the legs. Therefore, the flow of blood back to the heart is assisted by the massaging action on the veins of the skeletal muscles as they contract. This one-way flow of blood is ensured by the presence of *venous valves.*

Flow of Blood

The transportation of blood throughout the body is accomplished by the effort of two vascular systems: the arteries and the veins. Generally, veins have thinner walls than arteries and the blood in them is darker than that in arteries because it is oxygen poor. Blood is carried *to* the heart via the *veins.* Blood flows *away* from the heart by way of the *arteries.* The following is an overview of the circulation of blood in the body. Actually, the process is much more complex. It involves electrical impulses plus a system of valves and muscle tone. Throughout the synopsis, please refer to the general diagram showing flow of blood through arteries and veins, Figure 6-10, for orientation.

1. Blood enters the upper right-hand chamber of the heart, which is called the *right atrium.*
2. Contraction occurs in the right atrium, and the blood passes downward into a second chamber called the *right ventricle.*

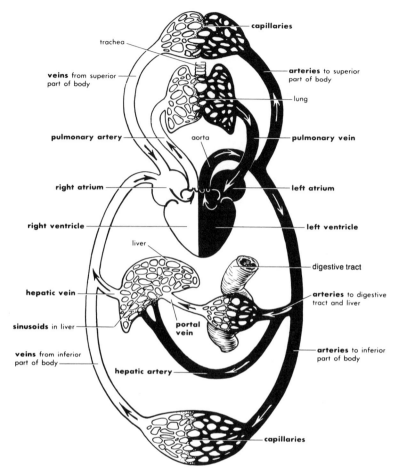

Fig. 6-10. Schematic representation of the double system of circulation. Oxygenated blood is shown in black; the nonoxygenated blood is white. The arrows indicate the direction of flow. (From Crouch, J. E.: Functional Human Anatomy, 4th Ed. Philadelphia, Lea & Febiger, 1985.)

3. Now the right ventricle contracts, forcing the blood into a large blood vessel called the *pulmonary artery.*
4. The pulmonary artery carries the blood to the lungs where carbon dioxide is exchanged for fresh oxygen. Now the blood is oxygen-rich and bright red.
5. The blood now flows from the lungs back to the heart through the *pulmonary veins.*
6. The pulmonary veins route the blood into the left upper chamber of the heart, which is called the *left atrium.*
7. Contraction of the left atrium pushes the blood into the most muscular chamber of the heart, the *left ventricle.*
8. Contraction of this chamber forces the blood into a large vessel called the *aorta.*

9. The aorta branches into subordinate arteries, which continue to divide and subdivide throughout the body until they become exceedingly small. The smallest arteries are called *arterioles.*
10. The arterioles subdivide into *capillaries,* which are thin-walled, microscopic pathways that connect with the veins.
11. It is to the blood in the capillaries that the tissues give up carbon dioxide and waste products in exchange for oxygen and nutrients. This causes the blood to change from bright red to a darker hue.
12. The capillaries now lead into tiny veins called *venules.* The venules lead into progressively larger veins, which in turn lead into major *veins.*
13. The major veins now carry the blood to the two veins that return the blood to the right atrium of the heart—the *superior* and *inferior vena cava.* The cycle begins again.

BASIC COAGULATION

Coagulation is defined by Dorland's Medical Dictionary as "the process of changing into a clot." Coagulation, or clotting, of blood is the action of three distinct components: (1) blood vessels, (2) blood platelets, and (3) coagulation factors. The collective action of the blood vessels and platelets in coagulation is known as primary hemostasis.

The blood vessels constitute the body's first line of defense. In response to various stimuli, the vessels contract at the site of injury. This causes a decrease in the blood flow and an aggregation of platelets.

Platelets are small cells that are normally found in the peripheral blood (Fig. 6-11). In addition to the role they play in coagulation, they also aid in the support of uninjured endothelial tissue. The platelets form a "plug" by adhering to the injured tissue. During this process, the platelets release their contents. These contents are called aggregating agents and are very powerful. Besides attracting more platelets to the injured site, these agents also elicit further contraction of the blood vessels and are involved in the activation of the coagulation factors. A lack of platelet function or a decreased number of circulating platelets will affect the delicately balanced hemostatic scheme. As

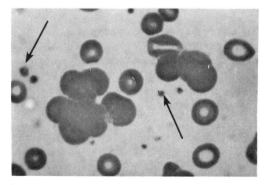

Fig. 6-11. Photograph of platelets. (From Brown, B. A.: Hematology: Principles and Procedures, 4th Ed. Philadelphia, Lea & Febiger, 1984.)

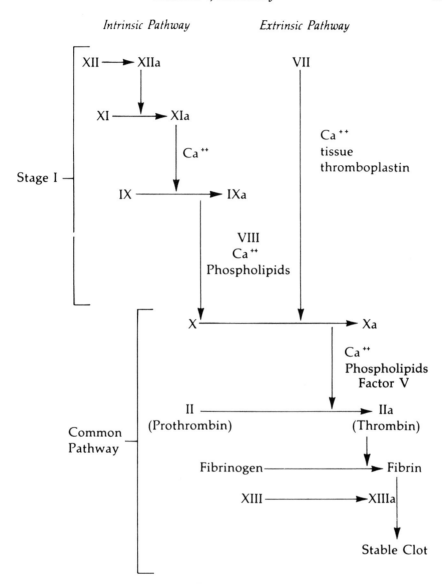

Fig. 6-12. The cascade concept of coagulation.

noted earlier, they are vital to the plug formation in vascular injury and in supplying phospholipids to the intrinsic pathway. The two primary tests for platelet activity are the *bleeding time,* which is used to assess platelet function, and the *platelet count,* which evaluates platelet production.

The production of the fibrin clot, which requires "coagulation factors," is known as secondary hemostasis. Secondary hemostasis has two pathways, the intrinsic and the extrinsic. These two pathways eventually join to form a common pathway, leading to the formation of a fibrin clot.

Each coagulation factor is assigned a Roman numeral, and the interaction of these factors has led to the "cascade" or "waterfall" concept (see Figure 6-12). The nomenclature for these coagulation factors has been established by the International Committee on Nomenclature of Blood Clotting Factors.

The activation of Factor XII initiates the intrinsic pathway. Now the system must go through a series of discrete activation steps before forming plasma thromboplastin. Factor XII converts Factor XI to the activated state. Now the activated Factor XI (XIa) in the presence of calcium ions enzymatically activates Factor IX (IXa). Activated Factor IX appears to form a complex with Factor VIII (antihemophilic factor), calcium ions, and phospholipids to activate Factor X. It is with Factor X that the common pathway begins.

The extrinsic pathway is activated when the blood (plasma) is exposed to a protein released by injured tissue and called tissue thromboplastin. In fact, the extrinsic pathway is able to bypass the discrete activation steps (known as stage I) in the intrinsic pathway because injured tissue supplies the thromboplastin directly to the system. In the extrinsic pathway, Factor VII, forming a complex with tissue thromboplastin and calcium ions, also activates Factor X.

From this point, the process is known as the "common pathway." Factor X, activated by both the Factor IX complex and the Factor VII complex, converts Factor II (prothrombin) into thrombin (IIa). Thrombin, in turn, cleaves the fibrinogen molecule. This alters the fibrinogen molecule so that it forms a fibrin clot, which is stabilized by Factor XIII.

Several tests are used to assess secondary hemostasis. The two most common ones are the activated partial thromboplastin time (APTT) and the prothrombin time (PT). The APTT is used to screen for deficiencies of the clotting factors in the intrinsic pathway; the PT is used to evaluate the extrinsic pathway.

Once healing has occurred and the blood vessel has repaired itself, the clot must be removed. This is done by the fibrinolytic mechanism known as fibrinolysis. Plasma contains a substance known as plasminogen. Activation of the coagulation system results in the conversion of plasminogen into the protease plasmin. Plasmin removes the clot by breaking fibrin down into smaller and smaller fragments known as fibrin-split products. In addition to the removal of clots, the fibrinolytic system keeps the vascular network free of deposited fibrin or fibrin clots.

BIBLIOGRAPHY

1. Anthony, C. P., and Thibodeau, G. A.: Textbook of Anatomy and Physiology. St. Louis, C. V. Mosby, 1979.
2. Barber, J.: Basic coagulation. Lab. Med., *9*:40, 1978.
3. Bick, R. L.: Clinical significance of fibrino (geno)-lytic degradation products (FDP) testing. Lab Lore, *9*:681, 1981.
4. Boggs, D. R., and Winkelstein, A.: White Cell Manual, 4th Ed. Philadelphia, F. A. Davis, 1983.
5. Brown, B. A.: Hematology: Principles and Procedures, 5th Ed. Philadelphia, Lea & Febiger, 1988.
6. Diggs, L. W., Strum, D., and Bell, A.: The Morphology of Human Blood Cells. North Chicago, Abbott Laboratories, 1978.
7. Finch, C. A.: Red Cell Manual. Seattle, University of Washington, 1969.

8. Fox, S. I.: Human Physiology. Dubuque, IA, Wm. C. Brown, 1984.
9. Graninick, H. R.: Intravascular coagulation 1. Differential diagnosis and conditioning mechanisms. Postgrad. Med., *62*:68, 1977.
10. Hillman, R. S., and Finch, C. A.: Red Cell Manual, 5th Ed. Philadelphia, F. A. Davis, 1985.
11. McKenzie, S. B.: Textbook of Hematology. Philadelphia, Lea & Febiger, 1988.
12. Steinberg, D.: Disseminated intravascular coagulation. Am. J. Med. Tech., *39*:392, 1973.
13. Tortora, G. J., and Anagnostakos, N. P.: Principles of Anatomy and Physiology, 4th Ed. New York, Harper & Row, 1984.

Chapter 7

THE BLOOD COLLECTION SYSTEM

DIAGRAMS OF EQUIPMENT

Evacuated Blood Collection System

This system, which is the most widely used system for collecting blood samples (see Figures 7-1–7-3), consists of a collection needle, a holder, and an evacuated glass tube containing a premeasured vacuum.

Nonevacuated Blood Collection System—Syringe

This system, although not used as extensively as the evacuated blood collection system, remains an important system for the collection of blood samples. It is primarily used in the microbiology section for the collection of blood cultures and on those individuals whose veins are difficult to stick. Like the evacuated blood collection system, this system is both entirely sterile and disposable. As noted in Figure 7-4, the syringe consists of a barrel (which is graduated into fractions of a milliliter) and a plunger. The needle (Fig. 7-5), which is packaged similarly to the evacuated blood collection system needle, is designed so that the hub will attach to a syringe and, thus, is not interchangeable with the evacuated blood collection system.

Figure 7-6 illustrates the different types of needle attachments found on syringes. The needle is fitted on the syringe by simply sliding the hub of the needle over the tip or Luer. The syringe on the right represents the Luer-Lok tip or "female-Luer." Slide the needle over the Luer and then give it a twist to hold it in place on the syringe. The advantage of the "male-Luer" is that the needle can be removed easily and quickly. This advantage may sometimes become a disadvantage, however, in that the needle can be removed from the syringe too easily and at the wrong time. The disadvantage of the "male-Luer" is the advantage of the "female-Luer," in that once properly attached, the needle stays on the syringe. This advantage can sometimes become a

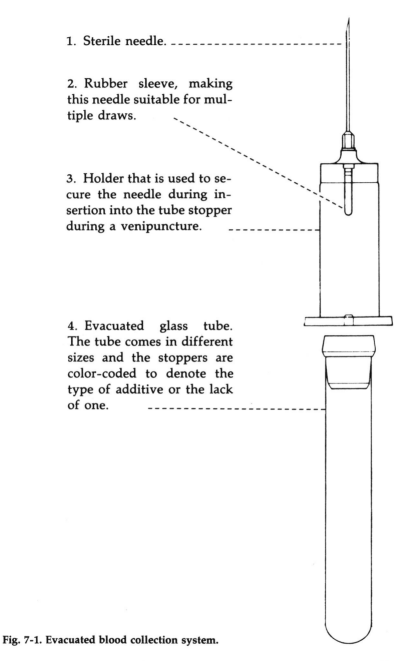

1. Sterile needle. _

2. Rubber sleeve, making this needle suitable for multiple draws.

3. Holder that is used to secure the needle during insertion into the tube stopper during a venipuncture. _ _ _ _ _ _ _ _ _ _ _

4. Evacuated glass tube. The tube comes in different sizes and the stoppers are color-coded to denote the type of additive or the lack of one. _

Fig. 7-1. Evacuated blood collection system.

problem in that occasionally it may be difficult to remove the needle. Another problem that might occur is the introduction of air bubbles into the blood sample if the needle is not properly attached.

5. Single-sample needle (Fig. 7-2). Note absence of rubber sleeve, exposing the short end of the needle, which punctures the rubber stopper.

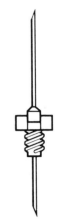

Fig. 7-2. Single-sample needle.

6. Sterile needles used with the evacuated system are available in peel-apart packages or plastic cases (as shown in Figure 7-3) and in different lengths (e.g., 1 inch, 1½ inches) and gauges (e.g., 20, 21, 22). The shields are color-coded for quick gauge identification.

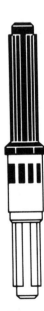

Fig. 7-3. Coded plastic case containing sterile needle.

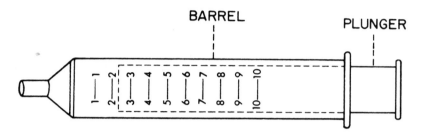

Fig. 7-4. Syringe. (From Brown, B.A.: Hematology: Principles and Procedures, 4th Ed. Philadelphia, Lea & Febiger, 1984.)

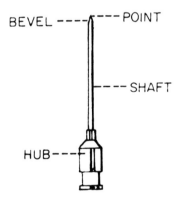

Fig. 7-5. Hypodermic needle. (From Brown, B.A.: Hematology: Principles and Procedures, 4th Ed. Philadelphia, Lea & Febiger, 1984.)

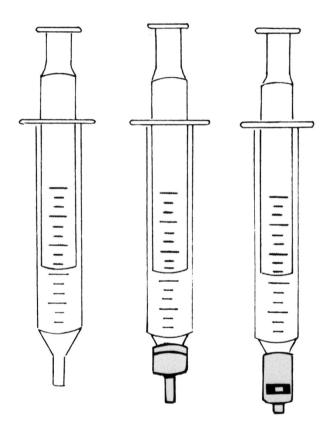

Fig. 7-6. The different types of needle attachments found on syringes. See text for explanation.

Monovette System

This blood collection system, developed by Sarstedt, is a combination of the syringe principle and the vacuum technique. Like other evacuated blood collection systems, the Monovette is color-coded and available with or without a variety of anticoagulants. To use it as a vacuum tube, pull the piston back until it clicks into the base. The piston rod can now be either unscrewed or broken off and discarded (Fig. 7-7). If, however, the venipuncture is difficult and a syringe would better serve the purpose, the Monovette can be filled by pulling back the piston. Multiple samples can be made by removing the Monovette from the guide-sleeve. The Monovette needle remains in the vein. On withdrawal of the Monovette, the rubber sleeve seals the free end of the needle (Fig. 7-8). Additional Monovettes can then be fitted into the guide-sleeve to continue the collection.

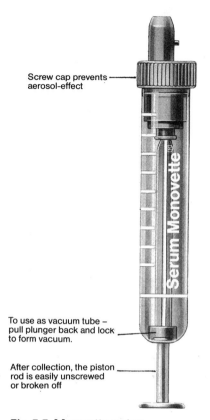

Screw cap prevents aerosol-effect

To use as vacuum tube – pull plunger back and lock to form vacuum.

After collection, the piston rod is easily unscrewed or broken off

Fig. 7-7. Monovette system.

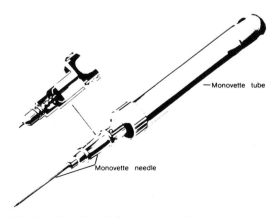

—Monovette tube

Monovette needle

Fig. 7-8. Details of Monovette needle.

Disposable Blood Lancets

A blood lancet (Fig. 7-9) is used for the collection of blood specimens by skin puncture. Blood lancets come in a variety of styles and point lengths. Some are plastic with metal tips. The lancet shown here is all metal and is available in individually sealed sterile packages.

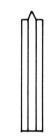

Fig. 7-9. Blood lancet.

Recently introduced is the Safety Flow Lancet (Fig. 7-10). Its concept is similar to that of the spring-loaded fingerstick devices except that once used, the entire mechanism is discarded. The blade remains within the holder until the button is pressed. Blade retraction is automatic on completion of the skin puncture. The blade is designed to create a wider puncture at the juncture of the dermal and subcutaneous tissue with minimal trauma. Three puncture depths are available: 1.4, 1.9, and 2.2 mm. The lancets are color coded according to puncture depth.

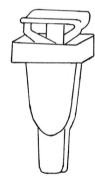

Fig. 7-10. Safety Flow lancet.

The Tenderfoot (Fig. 7-11) is a spring-loaded skin puncture device. However, after use it is disposable and cannot be reused. A safety clip is removed and the trigger is pushed. A pointed surgical steel blade then makes a horizontal sweeping motion and terminates in complete vertical blade retraction. An incision 1.0 mm in depth and 2.5 mm in length is made rather than a puncture wound. The blade depth is designed to make the incision above the major pain fibers and yet make for cleaner, freer blood flow.

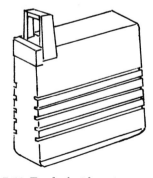

Fig. 7-11. Tenderfoot lancet.

Like the Tenderfoot, the Tenderlett (Fig. 7-12) is a disposable spring-loaded skin puncture device. It is designed for fingertip blood sampling and contoured to the shape of the finger to minimize skin indentation. Three incision depths and lengths are presently available: 1.75 mm $\times$ 0.94 mm for adults, 1.25 mm $\times$ 0.67 mm for pediatric patients, and 0.85 mm $\times$ 0.46 mm for infants and toddlers.

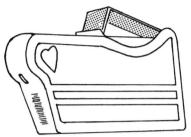

Fig. 7-12. Tenderlett lancet.

Spring-Loaded Skin Puncture Devices

On the market today are several reusable spring-loaded skin puncture devices for capillary blood sampling. Three examples are shown, the Autolet (Fig. 7-13), the Hemalet (Fig. 7-14), and the Monojector (Fig. 7-15). Their purpose is to make obtaining a capillary sample less frightening, faster, and a little less painful, and to keep skin damage to an absolute minimum. All have two main components: the disposable lancet and the finger platform or end cap. Hepatitis B virus outbreaks have been associated with the improper use of these devices for the collection of capillary blood specimens. To avoid this hazard, it is important that the lancet and the platform be replaced after each use.

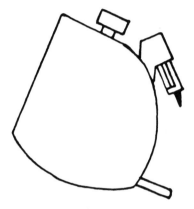

Fig. 7-13. Autolet.

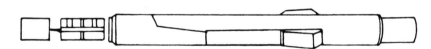

Fig. 7-14. Hemalet.

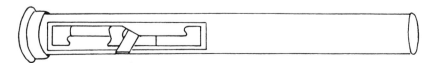

Fig. 7-15. Monojector.

Microtainer

The Microtainer (Fig. 7-16) is a single-tube, skin puncture collection device. It is available with or without a separator gel for serum collection, dipotassium EDTA or heparin for whole blood collection, and a glycolytic inhibitor. Also available is an amber Microtainer with separator gel. This amber tube protects specimens from virtually all ultraviolet light, helping to ensure the accuracy of photosensitive tests. A sample can be collected directly into the tube using the widemouth FloTop Collector. The Microtainers with additives have interior flow lines that channel the droplets of blood into the tube and provide reliable mixing without the need for beads. A special coating on the interior walls also helps the blood to reach the anticoagulant quickly and thus reduces the possibility of microclots. A new color-coded attachable plug may be securely fitted on the bottom of the tube. After specimen collection, the FloTop Collector is discarded and the plug is inserted on the top of the tube.

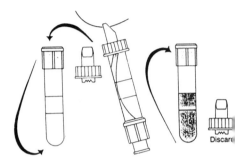

Fig. 7-16. Microtainer with FloTop Collector.

StatSampler

The StatSampler (Fig. 7-17) is assembled before use by inserting the capillary tube through the split stopper of the microtube. The microtube may contain a barrier gel, depending on its intended use. Capillary blood is then collected in a capillary tube that may or may not be coated with EDTA or heparin. After the blood is collected the assembly of capillary and microtube is turned to the vertical position, allowing the blood to drain into the microtube in which it can be rapidly separated for the preparation of plasma or serum, or used as whole blood.

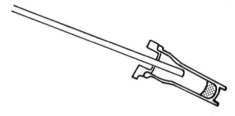

Fig. 7-17. StatSampler.

UNOPETTE System

The UNOPETTE system (Fig. 7-18) is designed for the preparation of micro blood specimens for use in hematology. It provides standardized procedures for collection, pipetting, and dilution. Each unit has a premeasured, prefilled reagent reservoir. The reservoir is equipped with a capillary pipette protected by a bullet-shaped shield. Most laboratories use this system to do manual platelet and reticulocyte counts, although other procedures are available.

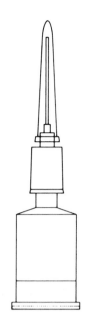

Fig. 7-18. UNOPETTE system.

Sarstedt Capillary Blood Collection System

These devices are intended for the collection of capillary blood, ranging from a maximum of 300 μl (Fig. 7-19) to 1 ml (Fig. 7-20). The device in Figure 7-19 consists of a sample tube and sample-tube holder. The specimen is collected by placing the sample tube into the blood. When filled, a small cap is attached to the narrow opening of the tube and it is placed in the holder. The device in Figure 7-20 is composed of a collection tube and a capillary unit. The tip of the capillary unit is placed in the blood, and the collection tube is allowed to fill. Both devices may be obtained with or without a variety of anticoagulants.

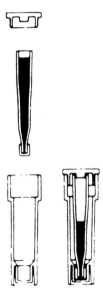

Fig. 7-19. Sarstedt 300 μl capillary blood collection system.

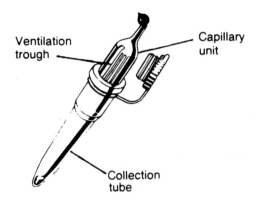

Fig. 7-20. Sarstedt 1 ml capillary blood collection system.

HOW THE PRIMARY ANTICOAGULANTS WORK

An anticoagulant prevents the blood from clotting by removing or neutralizing one of the essential factors necessary for coagulation. The anticoagulants routinely used in the clinical laboratory either (1) precipitate calcium, (2) bind calcium, or (3) inhibit thrombin.

Precipitate Calcium. Ammonium, lithium, potassium, or sodium oxalate prevents the coagulation of blood by removing calcium ions by precipitation as insoluble calcium oxalate. Using potassium oxalate as an example, the general or empiric formula is as follows:

$$K_2C_2O_4 \cdot H_2O + Ca \rightarrow \underline{CaC_2O_4} + K^{++}$$

A mixture of ammonium and potassium oxalate (double oxalate) is available primarily for use in Wintrobe sedimentation rates. Also, sodium oxalate is sometimes used in coagulation studies. However, the oxalates cause crenation of the red blood cells and bizarre forms of lymphocytes and monocytes, making them unsatisfactory for routine hematology procedures.

Bind Calcium. Ethylenediaminotetraacetic acid (EDTA), sodium polyanethole sulfonate (SPS), and sodium citrate prevent coagulation by binding calcium. EDTA and SPS are chelating agents. Chelation involves the bonding of a metal (in this case calcium) to a molecule that has two or more polar groups (the amine and carboxy groups in EDTA as illustrated in the empiric formula below). When this happens, a complex molecule is formed, removing the availability of calcium for the coagulation process.

Text continues on p. 66.

RUBBER STOPPER COLOR CODING*

Color	Characteristic	Volume of Draw	Concentration of Additive	Minimum Volume of Blood for Accurate Results
Red	No additives (for collection of serum)	2 to 20 ml	—	Not affected
Red & Gray	Polymer gel and clot activator (for collection of serum)	2.5 to 13 ml	—	Not affected
Lavender	Contains EDTA (for the collection of whole blood)	3 ml 7 ml 4 ml 7 ml	7.5% liquid K_3 15% liquid K_3 5.5 mg powder Na_2 10.5 mg powder Na_2	2 ml 5 ml Not affected Not affected
Green	Contains heparin (for the collection of whole blood)	2 to 10 ml	$14.3 \times$ tube size = USP Units	Not affected
Blue	Contains buffered sodium citrate (for coagulation studies)	1.8 to 4.5 ml	$0.105\ M$ (3.2%) or $0.129\ M$ (3.8%)	Full draw
Gray	Contains anticoagulant and glycolytic inhibitor (for glucose determinations)	3 to 10 ml	5 ml contains 10 mg potassium oxalate, 12.5 mg sodium fluoride; 10 ml contains 20 mg potassium oxalate, 25 mg sodium fluoride	Not affected
Yellow	Contains acid citrate dextrose (ACD) solution (for preservation of red blood cells) or sodium polyanethole sulfonate (SPS) (for blood culture specimens)	8.5 ml 4.2 ml 16.6 ml	1.5 ml 0.8 ml 3.4 ml	Not affected

*Available are evacuated tubes with rubber stoppers covered by a plastic shield. With a few exceptions, the color coding is similar to that of the rubber stoppers.

PRIMARY ANTICOAGULANTS AND THEIR ACTION

Anticoagulant	Action	Advantages/Disadvantages
1. EDTA (dipotassium salt of ethylenediaminetetraacetic acid)	Removes calcium by forming insoluble or un-ionized calcium salts, thereby preventing coagulation	Prevents platelet clumping and the formation of artifacts, therefore good for the preparation of blood films.
2. Sodium oxalate	As above	
3. Ammonium and potassium oxalate	As above	Cannot be used for blood films. Causes crenation of RBCs, bizarre forms of lymphs and monos.
4. Sodium citrate	As above	Anticoagulant of choice for coagulation studies because it protects certain of the procoagulants.
5. Heparin	Inactivates thrombin and thromboplastin	Unsatisfactory for blood smears because it causes background staining. Anticoagulant of choice for osmotic fragility tests because it does not affect the size of the red cells.

OTHER ADDITIVES AND THEIR ACTIONS

Additives	General Action
1. ACD solution (sodium citrate, citric acid, dextrose)	Red cell preservative
2. AD solution (citric acid, dextrose)	Red cell preservative
3. Alsever's solution	Red cell preservative
4. Buffered citrate (citric acid, sodium citrate)	Anticoagulant
5. CPD solution (sodium citrate, citric acid, sodium phosphate)	Red cell preservative
6. Sodium fluoride	Antiglycolytic agent
7. Lithium heparin	Anticoagulant
8. Lithium oxalate	Anticoagulant
9. Siliceous earth	Clotting activator
10. Sodium polyanethol sulfonate (SPS)	Anticoagulant (also inactivates complement, inhibits phagocytosis, reduces activity of certain antibiotics)
11. Sorbic acid	Antimycotic agent
12. Soybean meal (trypsin inhibitor)	Enzyme inhibitor
13. Thrombin	Clotting activator
14. Thymol	Antibacterial agent

TROUBLESHOOTING AND THE EVACUATED BLOOD COLLECTION SYSTEM

Problem Solving

General Problems	Possible Causes	Action
1. Short draw	Missed or transfixed vein	Redraw specimen if vein cannot be located
	Incomplete filling of tube	Allow tube to draw specified amount, thereby exhausting the vacuum
		Check vacuum by filling another tube with water
		Use tubes before expiration date
2. Tube breakage during centrifugation	Unbalanced centrifuge	Balance centrifuge before use by using shields matched by weight
3. Hemolyzed specimen	Traumatized specimen	Redraw specimen with a trauma-free venipuncture
4. Poor (mushy) clot formation or poor clot retraction	Insufficient clotting time	Allow specimen to clot completely
5. Presence of fibrin strands in serum tubes	Insufficient clotting time	Allow specimen to clot completely before centrifugation
6. Clotting in whole-blood (plasma) tubes	Insufficient mixing of additive with specimen	Mix well by inversion; make sure additive is not trapped around stopper by tapping tube lightly before filling
7. Stopper pop-off during mixing of whole-blood tubes before repeat testing	Positive pressure created by reinserting stopper	Vent tube while reinserting stopper
8. Incomplete barrier formation	Insufficient G force	Check centrifuge speed to make sure centrifuge is properly set to achieve force of 1200 G
9. Peel-back of barrier	Use of angle-head centrifuge	Decant serum after centrifugation or use swing-head centrifuge

Problem Solving

General Problems	Possible Causes	Action
EDTA		
10. False low hematocrit	Presence of excess EDTA owing to short draw	Check vacuum (see No. 1)
11. Cell distortion or hemolysis	Presence of excess EDTA caused by short draw or traumatic venipuncture	Check vacuum (see No. 1); redraw specimen with a trauma-free venipuncture
12. False low white cell and platelet count	Clotted specimen	Mix specimen well by inversion (see No. 6)
Citrate and Oxalate		
13. Prolonged coagulation time	Short draw High hematocrit, as in polycythemia; the small amount of plasma in such samples is inadequate to bind the available citrate	Check vacuum (see No. 1) to draw specified amount; use a reduced amount of anticoagulant
14. Low Westergren sedimentation rate	Incorrect ratio of citrate to specimen	Use tube with appropriate ratio of citrate to blood volume (1:4 recommended)
Heparin		
15. High sodium values	Sodium heparin salt interference	Use lithium heparin
16. High lithium values	Lithium heparin salt interference	Use sodium heparin
17. High BUN values	Ammonium heparin salt interference	Use lithium heparin

EDTA, which is also known as sequestrene and versene, is available as a free acid and as the di-, tri-, or tetra-salt. It is recommended that the potassium salt be used in preference to the sodium salt because of its greater solubility. EDTA is used perhaps more than any other anticoagulant for hematologic procedures. SPS, which is a weak chelating agent, is primarily used in the collection of blood cultures.

Sodium citrate also binds calcium by forming a soluble complex. Its effect is easily reversible by the addition of calcium. Consequently, it is the anticoagulant of choice for coagulation studies. In addition, it appears to preserve labile procoagulants. The general formula for the binding of calcium by sodium citrate is given below:

$$
\begin{array}{ccc}
\text{H—O} & & \text{H—O} \\
\text{H—C—C—O—Na} & & \text{H—C—C} \\
\text{O} & & \text{O \ O} \\
\text{HO—C—C—O—Na+Ca} \rightarrow & \text{HO—C—C—O—Ca} \\
\text{O} & & \text{O \ O} \\
\text{H—C—C—O—Na} & & \text{H—C—C} \\
\text{H} & & \text{H}
\end{array}
$$

Inhibit Thrombin. Heparin is available as an ammonium, lithium, or sodium salt, and its action is thought to prevent the transformation of prothrombin to thrombin and thus not allow a fibrin clot to form. It is a good anticoagulant because it causes the least interference in clinical chemistry tests. Unfortunately, it is expensive. In addition, it is not recommended for the preparation of blood smears when using Wright's stain because it causes a blue background to form on the smear.

SAFETY DEVICES

With the advent of the acquired immunodeficiency syndrome (AIDS) and the subsequent regulations and recommended guidelines by governmental and professional organizations covering the protection of health care professionals, a number of safety devices peculiar to blood collection have been developed. Three needle adapters are now on the market that have been designed to minimize the risk of needle stick injury following a venipuncture. When sampling is complete, the Saf-T Clik's (Fig. 7-21) outer sheath is slid

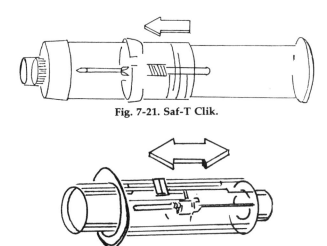

Fig. 7-21. Saf-T Clik.

Fig. 7-22. Acci-Guard.

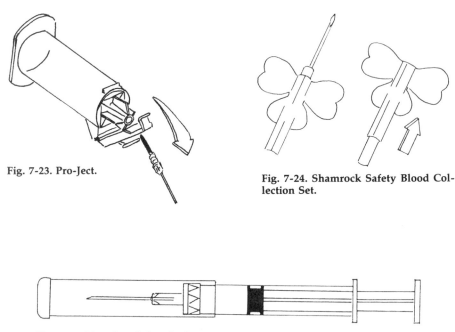

Fig. 7-23. Pro-Ject.

Fig. 7-24. Shamrock Safety Blood Collection Set.

Fig. 7-25. Monoject Safety Syringe.

forward over the exposed contaminated needle until a distinctive "click" is heard, indicating that the outer sheath is locked in place. The entire adapter may now be properly discarded and is not intended for reuse. The Acci-Guard (Fig. 7-22) is similar except that it is intended for limited reuse. By lightly pressing and gently sliding a tab back into the lock position, the needle is retracted into the adapter. A needle shield is dropped over the used needle through the front opening. The tab is then slowly moved forward until the covered needle is exposed. The covered needle is carefully twisted off and properly disposed. The Pro-Ject needle adapter (Fig. 7-23) is also designed for reuse. The adapter is placed over a biohazard container and the needle ejection lever is pushed forward using the thumb. The needle will be released, allowing it to fall into the biohazard container. Two other safety devices available are the Shamrock Safety Blood Collection Set (Fig. 7-24) and the Monoject Safety Syringe (Fig. 7-25). In both products, after blood collection is complete, the needle may simply be pulled into a protective shield that is locked into place.

TUBE AND HOLDER SIZE

Figure 7-26 illustrates the most commonly employed evacuated tubes and the proper size of holder to use with the tubes. Given with each tube is the amount of blood that is supposed to be drawn.

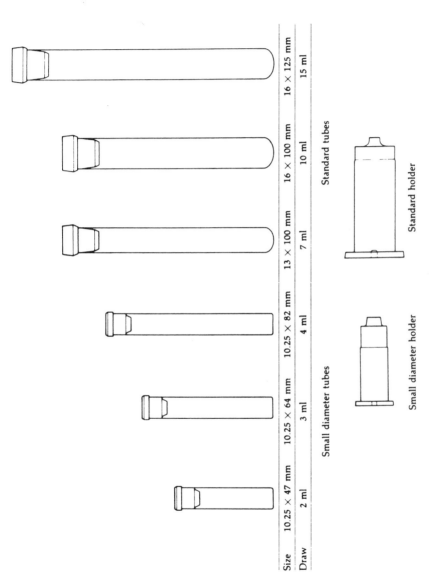

Size	10.25 × 47 mm	10.25 × 64 mm	10.25 × 82 mm	13 × 100 mm	16 × 100 mm	16 × 125 mm
Draw	2 ml	3 ml	4 ml	7 ml	10 ml	15 ml

Small diameter tubes

Standard tubes

Small diameter holder

Standard holder

Fig. 7-26. Commonly employed evacuated tubes.

BIBLIOGRAPHY

1. A Guide to the VACUTAINER Brand Evacuated Blood Collection System. Rutherford, NJ, Becton Dickinson Co., 1976.
2. Acci-guard Reusable Blood Collection Holder, Product Information. Denver, CO, Medical Safety Products, 1990.
3. Autolet Product Information. Oxford, England, Owen Mumford, Ltd., 1981.
4. Brown, B. A.: Hematology: Principles and Procedures, 5th Ed. Philadelphia, Lea & Febiger, 1988.
5. Calam, R. R. (Chairholder): Procedures for the Handling and Processing of Blood Specimens. Villanova, PA, National Committee for Clinical Laboratory Standards, 1990.
6. Capillary Blood Collection-CB 1000/CB 300, Product Information. Princeton, NJ, W. Sarstedt, 1982.
7. Hemalet, Product Information. New York, Medprobe Laboratories, 1982.
8. Henry, R. J., Cannon, D. C., and Winkelman, J. W. (eds.): Clinical Chemistry: Principles and Techniques, 2nd Ed. New York, Harper & Row, 1974.
9. Microtainer Brand Safety Flow Lancets, Product Information. Rutherford, NJ, Becton Dickinson Co., 1990.
10. Microtainer Brand Tubes, Product Information. Rutherford, NJ, Becton Dickinson Co., 1989.
11. Monoject Safety Syringe, Product Catalog. St. Louis, MO, Sherwood Medical, 1989.
12. Pro-Ject Safety Needle Holder, Product Information. El Toro, CA, Pro-Tec Containers, 1990.
13. Saf-T Click Shielded Blood Needle Adapter, Product Information. Brentwood, TN, Ryan Medical, 1990.
14. Shamrock Safety Blood Collection Set, Product Information. Brentwood, TN, Ryan Medical, 1990.
15. Shuna, Vera, Personal Communication, 1991.
16. StatSampler MicroBlood Collectors, Product Information. Norwood, MA, StatSpin Technologies, 1990.
17. Tenderfoot, Product Information. Edison, NJ, International Technidyne Corp., 1989.
18. Tenderlet, Product Information. Edison, NJ, International Technidyne Corp., 1991.
19. Tietz, N. W. (ed.): Fundamentals of Clinical Chemistry, 3rd Ed. Philadelphia, W. B. Saunders, 1987.
20. Whitaker, V. G.: Biohazard warning: HBV and spring-loaded fingerstick devices. Lab-Oratory, *58:*2, 1990.
21. Wiseman, J. D. (Chairholder): Devices for Collection of Skin Puncture Blood Specimens, 2nd Ed. Villanova, PA, National Committee for Clinical Laboratory Standards, 1990.
22. VACUTAINER Brand Systems, Product Catalog. Rutherford, NJ, Becton Dickinson Co., 1981.

Chapter **8**

PERFORMANCE OF A ROUTINE VENIPUNCTURE

PRINCIPLE

A patient's veins are the main source of blood for laboratory testing as well as a point of entry for IVs and blood transfusions. Since only a few veins are easily accessible to both laboratory and other medical personnel, it is important that everything be done to preserve their good condition and availability.

EQUIPMENT

1. Tourniquet
2. 70% alcohol prep pads
3. Dry gauze pads
4. Appropriate evacuated tubes for tests ordered
5. Evacuated blood collection system holder or syringe
6. Plastic adhesive pressure strip

PROCEDURE

1. Review the request form(s). See what test(s) have been ordered and that you have the appropriate evacuated tubes.
2. Be sure to knock on the patient's door before you enter the room.
3. Identify the patient. This is the *most important step* in the performance of a venipuncture.
   Note (3):
   (a) If the patient is conscious and competent, you may presumptively make an identification by asking him his full name.
   (b) Confirm the patient's identification by the armband, making sure that the name on the armband and that on the request form are identical.

71

(c) If the name on the request does not match the one on the armband or if no armband is present, have one of the nurses identify the patient. Note the nurse's name and the fact that she identified the patient on the request form.

4. Let the patient know that you are from the laboratory and that you need to collect a blood sample that the patient's physician has ordered.
Note (4):
Emphasize that the patient's physician has ordered the test(s). This underscores its importance and necessity.

5. Check for diet restrictions.
Note (5):
If the test requires that the patient be fasting, make sure that these requirements have been followed. Also, if the patient is to have nothing by mouth (NPO—nothing per os), you are not to give the patient anything to eat *or drink,* even if he asks for it.

6. Reassure the patient.
Note (6):
Gain the patient's confidence. *Never* say, "this won't hurt." Let him know that the venipuncture may be a little painful, but will be of short duration.

7. Properly position the patient.
Note (7):
(a) Have bed patients lie on their backs in a comfortable position. Do the same for any patient when you believe that the position would be safer for them or would make it easier for you to perform the procedure. Add support under the arm with a pillow if needed. Extend the arm so as to form a straight line from the shoulder to the wrist.
(b) Ambulatory patients or outpatients should be comfortably seated in a venipuncture chair. The arm should be positioned on a slanting armrest in a straight line from the shoulder to the wrist. The arm should not be bent at the elbow.
(c) Make sure the patient does not have anything in his mouth.
(d) NEVER do a venipuncture on a patient who is standing.

8. Prepare your equipment. Assemble your tube and needle holder, syringe and needle, gauze, plastic adhesive pressure strip, and 70% alcohol prep before you apply the tourniquet.

Note (8):
(a) Check the requisition form(s) again for tube verification.
(b) Select the proper size needle. The choice of needle usually depends on the size of the vein. The most frequently used needle in the majority of hospitals is the 21 gauge. Usually, the higher the gauge number, the smaller the diameter or bore; however, you may see advertised a 21-gauge needle with a 20-gauge draw. This means that the wall of the needle is thin enough so that the diameter of the needle can be equivalent to a 21-gauge and the bore to a 20-gauge. For extremely small veins, most venipuncturists will use the 22- to 23-gauge needle. The length of the needle (1 to 1½ inches) is an individual choice.
(c) The collection tray and assembled venipuncture equipment should be placed on a stand next to the patient, but *not* on the patient's bed.

9. Select site for venipuncture. DO NOT DRAW BLOOD ABOVE AN INTRAVENOUS INFUSION.
Note (9):
Application of Tourniquet (see Figures 8-1 through 8-4) Wrap the tourniquet around the arm approximately 3 to 4 inches above the area where you are going to "feel" for a vein (Fig. 8-1). Hold one end taut (Fig. 8-2). Then tuck a portion of the end under the taut end so as to form a loop

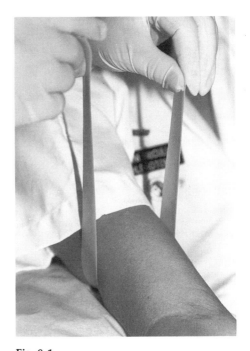

Fig. 8-1.

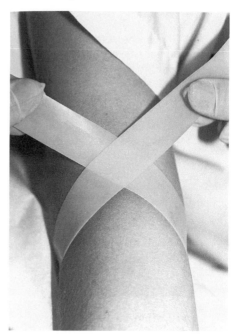

Fig. 8-2.

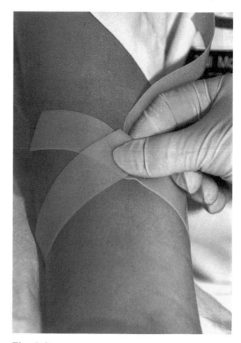

Fig. 8-3.

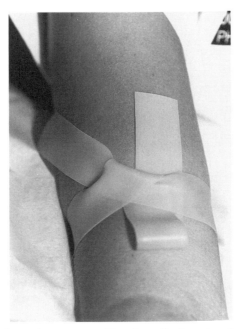

Fig. 8-4. Front view of tourniquet on arm. To release the tourniquet, carefully pull the end of the tourniquet on the left.

(Fig. 8-3). If applied correctly, the tourniquet should look similar to that in Figure 8-4.

Vein Selection

(a) The three veins primarily used for venipunctures are the cephalic, basilic, and median cubital (see Figure 8-5).

(b) Have the patient make a fist, which usually makes the veins more prominent; however, vigorous pumping should be avoided.

(c) Using the index finger, palpate (feel) for a vein. Even if you can see the vein, palpate so you can be certain of its location and direction. A vein feels much like an elastic tube and "gives" under pressure. Also, veins do not pulsate as arteries do. If you have difficulty finding a vein, if possible, examine the other arm. Sometimes veins in one arm will be larger than in the other. If the superficial veins of the arms are either impossible to find or not available, you may want to examine for veins in the wrist, hands, or feet. TAKE YOUR TIME, FIND THE BEST VEIN, BUT NEVER LEAVE THE TOURNIQUET ON FOR LONGER THAN *1 MINUTE.*

(d) Release the tourniquet before you clean the venipuncture site.

10. Clean venipuncture site.

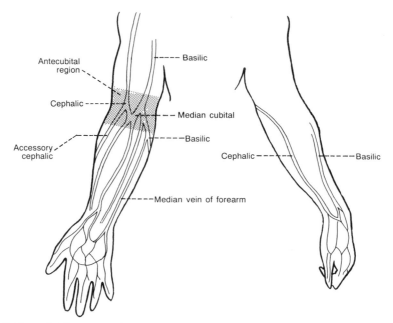

Fig. 8-5. Superficial veins of the right (anterior view) and left (posterior view) arms.

Note (10):
(a) Remove the alcohol prep from its sterile package.
(b) Cleanse the vein site with a circular motion from the center to the periphery.
(c) Allow the area to dry. You may fan the area with your hand but do not blow on the site.
(d) If the venipuncture is a difficult one and you have to palpate for the vein after you have cleansed the site, repeat the cleaning procedure.

11. Reapply tourniquet.
12. Grasp the patient's arm approximately 1 to 2 inches below the venipuncture site. Pull the skin tight with your thumb to keep the vein from rolling.
13. Perform the venipuncture.
Note (13):
(a) Insert the appropriate needle onto the syringe or thread the needle into the holder.
(b) If an evacuated tube is used, insert the tube into the holder and onto the needle up to the recessed guideline. Do not push pass this line because it will cause a loss of vacuum.
(c) The needle should be at approximately a 15° angle to the patient's arm and in a direct line with the vein (see Figure 8-6).

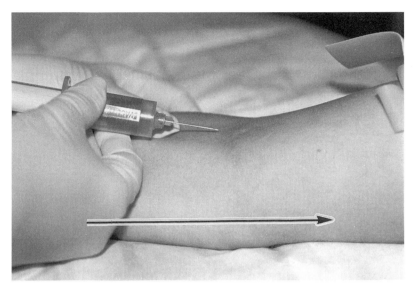

Fig. 8-6.

(d) The syringe or tube should be below the venipuncture site to prevent backflow, and the arm (or other venipuncture site) be placed in a downward position.

(e) Turn the needle so that the bevel is in an upward position.

(f) Puncture the vein. The puncture of the skin and vein should be done, if possible, in one motion.

(g) If a syringe is used, care must be taken not to pull on the plunger too rapidly or forcefully.

(h) If an evacuated tube is used, as soon as the needle enters the vein, push the tube as far as it will go.

(i) Steady the needle holder so that the needle is not inadvertently removed from the vein, causing a "short draw."

(j) If multiple samples are drawn, remove the tube as soon as the blood flow stops and insert the next tube into the holder.

(k) Those tubes with additives should be mixed immediately but gently.

14. Release the tourniquet.
Note (14):
The tourniquet may be released as soon as blood enters the tube, or you may leave the tourniquet on during the entire procedure.

15. Have the patient open his hand.
16. Place a square of sterile gauze over the puncture site and quickly remove the needle (see Figure 8-7).

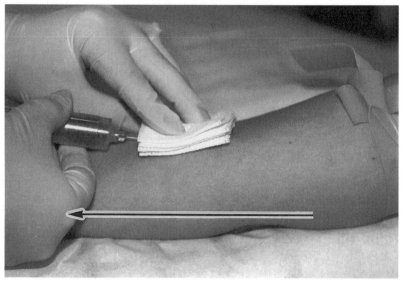

Fig. 8-7.

17. Apply pressure until the bleeding has stopped, then place a plastic adhesive pressure strip over the venipuncture site.
18. Label tubes as follows (minimum information):
    a. patient's name
    b. time specimen collected
    c. date
    d. initials of collector
19. WASH YOUR HANDS BEFORE STICKING THE NEXT PATIENT.
20. Before leaving the room, make sure you have removed all the used equipment and *thanked the patient.*

QUALITY ASSURANCE

1. Do not attempt to stick a patient more than two (2) times. See Chapter 12.
2. DO NOT STICK ABOVE AN IV. If an IV is running in both arms, and no other vein is available except in the area of the IV administration, specimens may be drawn *below* the IV site as follows: (1) With the attending physician's permission, have the nursing staff turn off the IV for no less than 2 minutes before venipuncture. (2) Apply the tourniquet *below* the IV site. A vein other than the one with the IV should be used. (3) After doing the venipuncture, draw 5 ml of blood. Discard this blood, *then* draw the blood sample to be used for testing.
3. Make sure that all blue top tubes have a "full draw." Partial draws will affect the coagulation results. If possible, always "draw" the blue top tube after you have "drawn" at least one other tube.
4. Label tubes *after* you have stuck the patient, NOT BEFORE.

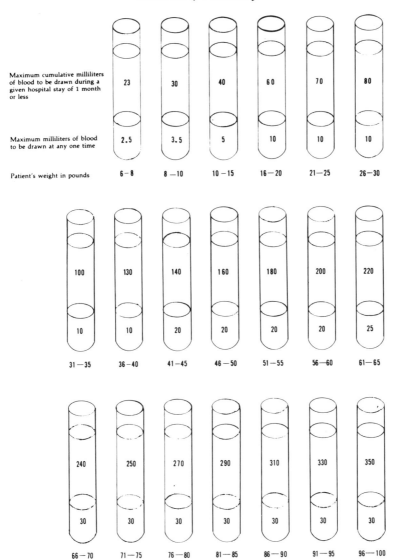

Fig. 8-8. Maximum milliliters of blood to be drawn from patients under 14 years of age. (Adapted from Becan-McBride, K.: Textbook of Clinical Laboratory Supervision. New York, Appleton-Century-Crofts, 1982.)

5. If you notice the venipuncture area beginning to swell while you are drawing the blood, immediately release the tourniquet, remove the needle, and apply pressure with the gauze square.

6. Do not keep the tourniquet on a patient's arm more than 1 minute.

7. Outpatients should be seated for approximately 15 minutes before a venipuncture is attempted.

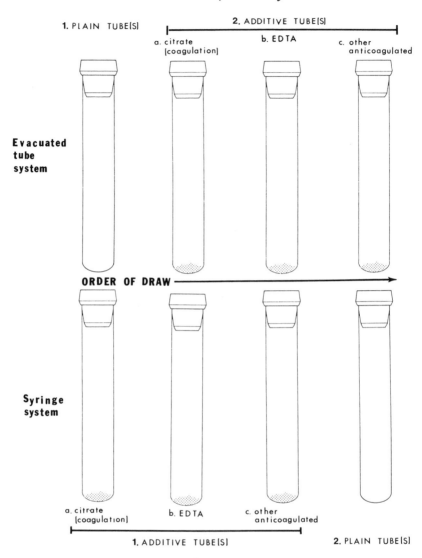

Fig. 8-9.

8. The order of tube draw is possibly important for obtaining accurate values. This is suggested especially when using the evacuated tube system, because there is a risk of contaminating a subsequent tube with the additive from a tube just collected. For example, if a tube containing the potassium salt of EDTA is collected prior to a tube for electrolyte evaluation, it is possible that the potassium value could be falsely increased. Likewise, the order in which blood is added to tubes when a syringe is used is important, because of the possibility of microclots, which can cause erroneous coagulation and hematologic results. The recommended order of draw is outlined in Figure 8-9. However, it is recommended that if

electrolyte levels are determined on plasma drawn in a green stopper tube containing lithium or ammonium heparin, and if coagulation studies or a complete blood count (CBC) is also ordered, the heparinized specimen should be collected before the citrated or EDTA tube to avoid possible sodium or potassium contamination. It has been suggested that a plain (red stopper) tube that contains a clot activator should be treated as an additive tube in the order of draw. Because of a lack of consensus, each health care institution must make its own decision regarding this matter.

BIBLIOGRAPHY

1. Becan-McBride, K. (ed.): Textbook of Clinical Laboratory Supervision. New York, Appleton-Century-Crofts, 1982.
2. Brown, B. A.: Hematology: Principles and Procedures, 5th Ed. Philadelphia, Lea & Febiger, 1988.
3. DaCunha, J. P., Ford, R. D., and Glover, S. M. (eds.): Diagnostics. Springfield, PA, Intermed. Comm., 1981.
4. Geller, Shayna, personal communication, 1991.
5. So You're Going to Collect A Blood Specimen. Skokie, IL, College of American Pathologists, 1974.
6. Statland, B. E.: Specimen collection and heparin. Med. Lab. Obser., *18:*16, 1986.
7. Statland, B. E., Boke, H., and Winkel, P.: Factors contributing to intra-individual variations of serum constituents: 4. Effects of posture and tourniquet application on variation of serum constituents in healthy subjects. Clin. Chem., *20:*1513, 1974.
8. Stockbower, J. M. (Chairman): Standard Procedures for the Collection of Diagnostic Blood Specimens by Venipuncture. Villanova, PA, National Committee on Clinical Laboratory Standards, 1977.

Chapter 9

PROCEDURE FOR A SKIN PUNCTURE

PRINCIPLE

Skin punctures may be used to collect blood on patients of all ages; however, the skin puncture technique is primarily used for adults on whom it is difficult to do a venipuncture and on infants. Meites and Levitt give two main reasons for collecting blood by skin punctures on infants: (a) microvolumes of blood are desirable to avoid anemia and (b) veins must be reserved for parenteral therapy.

EQUIPMENT

1. 70% alcohol prep pads
2. Dry gauze pads
3. Sterile lancet, with tips up to 5 mm long for older children and adults and tips 2.4 mm or less for newborns
4. Possibly, a heel-warming device
5. Capillary tubes and/or Microtainers
6. Glass microslides

PROCEDURE

1. Select the puncture site.
2. Warm the puncture site to increase the blood flow.
   Note (2):
   (a) Cover the area for 3 minutes with a towel that has been soaked in 39 to 44°C water.
   (b) OR, you may warm the area by using one of the commercial infant heel warmers.

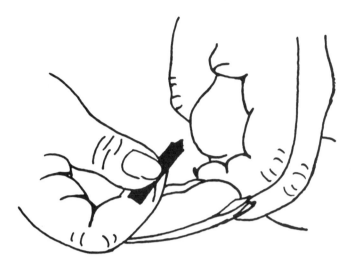

Fig. 9-1. Proper positioning for heel stick.

3. Clean the puncture site similarly to the procedure used when doing a venipuncture. After application of the alcohol, completely dry the area with a sterile gauze square. The presence of alcohol will quickly hemolyze the blood.

4. When doing a heel stick on an infant, hold the heel gently but firmly. This may be done in one of two ways: (1) place the forefinger around the ankle, and the thumb over the arch of the foot (see Figure 9-1), or (2) place the forefinger over the arch of the foot and the thumb below the puncture site at the ankle. Use only lancets with a maximum tip length of 2.4 mm. Make the puncture in one continuous, deliberate motion, perpendicular to the puncture site. Punctures should be made on the most medial or most lateral portion of the plantar surface (shaded areas in the diagram of an infant's foot, Figure 9-2). It is also recommended that you do not perform skin punctures on the posterior curvature of the heel.

   Note (4):
   The depth of the skin puncture in the heel is important in infants, particularly neonates. *It must not exceed 2.4 mm.* Penetration of the calcaneous bone, osteomyelitis, and sepsis have all been reported as potential complications.

5. For a finger stick, place your thumb above and well away from the puncture site. The procedure is similar to that for the heel. The stick should be made into the pulp of the finger (as shown in the shaded area in Figure 9-3) in one continuous motion. It should not be directed toward the bone. This will usually require a 10 to 20° angle to the longitudinal axis of the phalangeal bone.

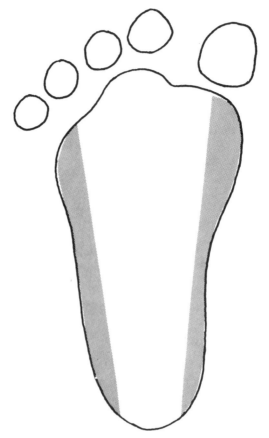

Fig. 9-2. Diagram showing the areas (shaded) of an infant's foot that may be used for skin puncture.

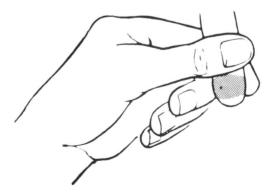

Fig. 9-3. Area of fingertip puncture. (Modified from Brown, B. A.: Hematology: Principles and Procedures, 4th Ed. Philadelphia, Lea & Febiger, 1984.)

Note (5):

The pain of a deep puncture is no more than that for a superficial one. Not only will you get a better flow of blood, but you may spare the patient from having to be stuck again.

6. Wipe away the first drop of blood, using a dry gauze, because it may be contaminated with tissue fluids.

7. Moderate pressure may be applied, but do not vigorously massage the area.

8. Collect the blood in the appropriate container.

9. Label the container as follows:
   a. patient's name
   b. time of collection
   c. date of collection
   d. initials of collector

QUALITY ASSURANCE

1. Do not stick a baby's heel more than twice to obtain a blood sample.

2. Make sure the area for the skin puncture is completely dry before carrying out the procedure.

3. Remember not to squeeze the finger too tightly so as to avoid diluting the blood with tissue juices.

4. Collect hematology specimens first, then chemistry and blood bank samples.

5. On the request form note that the specimen is from a skin puncture.

6. If the blood specimen is collected in capillary tubes, to avoid loss of any of the tubes or errors in identification, it is advisable to seal one end of the tubes and place them in a single large test tube. This can then be labeled with the patient's name and other pertinent information.

BIBLIOGRAPHY

1. Meites, S., and Levitt, M. J.: Skin-puncture and blood-collecting techniques for infants. Clin. Chem., *25*:183, 1979.
2. Phelan, S.: Blood Collection: The Pediatric Patient. Chicago, IL, ASCP Press, 1990.
3. Randolph, V. S.: Considerations for the clinical laboratory serving the pediatric patient. Am. J. Med. Tech., *48*:7, 1982.
4. Stockbower, J. M. (Chairman): Standard Procedure for the Collection of Diagnostic Blood Specimens by Skin Puncture. Villanova, PA, National Committee on Clinical Laboratory Standards, 1978.

Chapter 10

NURSERY TECHNIQUE

PRINCIPLE

Newborns and premature infants are at a high risk of infection because their immune systems are immature. Newborns become colonized with their mother's normal flora; however, they can pick up microorganisms from the personnel who work in the nursery. This can pose a potentially life-threatening situation.

EQUIPMENT

1. Clean gowns
2. Disposable masks
3. Handwashing facilities
4. Laboratory equipment for skin puncture

PROCEDURE

1. If required, place disposable booties over shoes.
2. Wash hands as described under Handwashing, Chapter 4.
3. Put on a clean gown and disposable mask. (Under certain situations, sterile gloves may also be required.)
4. Take into the nursery only those items needed to perform the skin puncture and collect the blood specimen. *Do not take the entire blood collection tray.*
5. After collection of the specimen, return to the anteroom to properly label all tubes.
6. Deposit gowns, masks, booties in the proper receptacles and *wash your hands.*

BIBLIOGRAPHY

1. Castle, M.: Hospital Infection Control, Principles and Practice. New York, John Wiley and Sons, 1980.
2. Soule, B. M. (ed.): The APIC Curriculum for Infection Control Practice, Vol. II. Dubuque, IA, Kendall/Hunt Publishing Co., 1983.

Chapter **11**

ARTERIAL PUNCTURES

Arterial punctures are now rarely performed by laboratory personnel. Arterial blood is used to evaluate gas exchange in the lungs by measuring the partial pressure of oxygen and carbon dioxide; therefore, this procedure is most often a function of the respiratory therapy department. Since some laboratories still do blood gases, however, the general techniques for doing arterial sticks have been included in this handbook. *It must be emphasized that an arterial puncture is a dangerous procedure. Only those individuals who have been extensively trained in the technique and who have been approved by the medical staff should attempt to do arterial punctures.*

1. The following equipment is generally standard for performing arterial punctures:
    a. a 2- to 5-ml syringe or collection device that is impermeable to gas exchange
    b. a rubber stopper
    c. heparin
    d. 20-gauge and 23-gauge needles
    e. an emesis basin or zip-lock plastic bag
    f. crushed ice

To prepare the syringe, first attach a 20-gauge needle to the syringe and draw approximately 1.0 ml of heparin into the barrel. Continuously rotate the barrel of the syringe while pulling back on the plunger. Make sure you pull the plunger back at least past the 3.0-ml mark. Now gently expel the heparin, again rotating the syringe. Remove the 20-gauge needle and aseptically attach the 23-gauge needle. Just before you attempt the arterial puncture, eject the remaining heparin.

2. Perform the Allen test to assess circulation. This is accomplished in the following manner:

a. Rest the patient's arm on the bedside table, supporting the wrist with a rolled towel. Have the patient clench his fist.

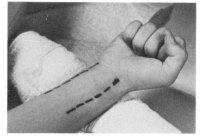

Fig. 11-1.

b. Using the middle and index fingers of each hand, exert pressure on both the radial and ulnar arteries.

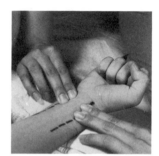

Fig. 11-2.

c. Without removing pressure, have the patient unclench his fist. Note the palm for blanching, which indicates impaired blood flow.

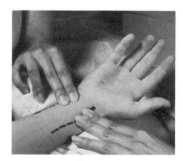

Fig. 11-3.

d. Release the pressure on the ulnar artery. Check to see whether the palm begins to turn pink in around 5 seconds. If it does not, this may indicate that there is possible occlusion of the radial artery or poor cardiac output. If this is the case, do the Allen test on the other wrist.

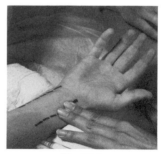

Fig. 11-4.

Note:

It is *important* when doing an arterial puncture that you be *very honest* with the patient. Explain what the procedure is and that it will be uncomfortable. Solicit the patient's cooperation, reminding him to remain still. *Do not promise that cooperation will guarantee success.*

3. When trying to locate an artery, constant pressure with the middle and index fingers is the method of choice, rather than palpating, as is done when trying to locate a vein.
4. Using a circular motion, clean the puncture site with a povidone-iodine solution. Next, wipe the area in the same manner, using 70% alcohol. Let the puncture site air dry. Do not blow on it. In the same manner, clean the fingers that will be used to locate the artery.
5. Locate the artery with one hand while holding the sampling device or syringe with the other.
6. Puncture the skin at a 45 to 60° angle. Advance the needle slowly. When you puncture an artery, the blood will "pulsate" into the collection device, pushing the plunger up of its own accord. *Never pull back on the plunger.*
7. Never attempt more than twice to do an arterial puncture, and *never probe.*
8. After you have obtained the sample, gently expel any air bubbles by holding the syringe in an upright position and slowly forcing a small amount of blood out of the syringe into a 2 × 2-inch gauze pad. Some collection devices are designed so that this problem does not occur.
9. Next, stick the needle into a rubber stopper to seal it from the air.
10. Mix the specimen gently but thoroughly.
11. Place the sample on ice for transportation to the laboratory.
12. After removing the needle, apply firm pressure to the puncture site for at least 5 minutes. After pressure is released, tape a bandage firmly over the puncture site. Do not, however, tape the entire wrist since this may restrict circulation.

Note:

Never ask the patient to apply the pressure. The patient may not apply pressure sufficiently or for a long enough time.

BIBLIOGRAPHY

1. DaCunha, J. P., Ford, R. D., and Glover, S. M. (eds.): Diagnostics. Springfield, PA, Intermed Communications, Inc., 1981.

Chapter 12

PROCEDURE WHEN UNABLE TO OBTAIN A BLOOD SPECIMEN

For any number of reasons, it may be impossible to obtain a blood specimen. The patient may be absent from the room, may refuse to be stuck, or may present difficulties in having a venipuncture performed. If any one of these situations occurs, the following general protocol should be followed.

PATIENT NOT IN ROOM

If, when going to do a venipuncture, the patient is not in the room, inform the nursing station and request that they call the laboratory as soon as the patient returns. Upon returning to the laboratory, report the situation to the appropriate supervisor.

PATIENT REFUSES TO ALLOW VENIPUNCTURE

If an adult patient refuses to be stuck, attempt gentle persuasion by reminding the patient that his physician needs the results of the laboratory tests to aid in the patient's recovery. *Never argue or get upset with the patient (or with the patient's family), and never subject the patient to any form of duress.*

If in a hospital situation, report the problem to the nursing station. Often, patients will respond to reasoning by the nurses when they will not listen to or cooperate with anyone else.

If the patient still refuses, report to the appropriate laboratory supervisor that the patient would not allow a venipuncture. Notify or have the nurses notify the attending physician of the situation. Document the refusal on the laboratory request. For an adolescent who refuses a venipuncture, the same procedure should be followed as for an adult—even if the parents give their permission for a venipuncture and offer their support.

If a child refuses to be stuck, the parents should be consulted. If the parents are willing and give their permission to attempt the venipuncture, their assistance in securing the child is not only physically supportive but also gives physical evidence of their consent. If the parents do not offer their assistance or give their permission, the appropriate individuals should be notified and the refusal noted on the laboratory request.

It is important to remember that when a child needs medical attention, particularly if admitted to the hospital, the parents may be distraught and even suffer from an unwarranted sense of guilt. Consequently, they might react belligerently toward anyone whom they perceive as inflicting additional and unnecessary pain on their child. It is important to be sensitive to their feelings and always be as tactful as possible.

DIFFICULT VENIPUNCTURE

Unfortunately, all veins are not large, prominent, and easy to stick. From time to time, even those best at performing venipunctures have difficulty in obtaining blood. If after palpating, you decide to attempt a venipuncture and you miss or for some reason cannot get any blood, try only once more.

If, after the second attempt, you still have not obtained a specimen, notify the nursing station and/or the appropriate laboratory supervisor of the problem. This is particularly important if it is a timed specimen (e.g., glucose tolerance).

The supervisor, or someone designated, will make a second attempt. Except in extenuating circumstances, this too should be limited to two tries. If a specimen is still not obtained, the nursing station and/or the physician are to be notified and the appropriate notations recorded.

Note:

It was noted in a previous section that if the veins in one arm do not appear suitable for venipuncture, the other arm should be examined. If it appears, however, that drawing blood from the veins in either arm would be difficult, other sites should be examined and considered. These include veins in the hands, legs, and feet. A WORD OF CAUTION: Venipunctures performed on the hands, feet, and legs are both difficult and potentially dangerous. The venipuncturist attempting to obtain blood from these sites must be knowledgeable regarding the proper techniques. The veins of the hands are not "fixed," so they have a tendency to roll and are difficult to stick. Also, an abundant supply of nerves is located in the hands. This not only makes venipunctures in the hands more uncomfortable for the patient, but in addition may cause potential complications because of nerve damage. Most often, venipunctures in the legs and feet are performed on the elderly. This group of patients frequently suffers from varicosity, resulting in venous stagnation; thus, venipuncture sites in these areas heal slowly. Both the hands and the feet are notoriously contaminated with bacteria. This greatly increases the chances of infection from any invasive technique.

BIBLIOGRAPHY

1. Laboratory Safety and Accident Manual. Valdosta, GA, Doctors Laboratory Inc., 1991.
2. Phlebotomy Procedure Manual. Rochester, MN, Mayo Clinic, 1986.
3. So You're Going to Collect a Blood Specimen. Skokie, IL, College of American Pathologists, 1974.

Chapter 13

PREPARATION OF A BLOOD SMEAR

Blood smears can be made from either capillary blood (fingerstick) or venous blood. The three procedures for preparing blood smears are (1) the spun smear, (2) the coverslip smear, and (3) the slide wedge smear. The slide wedge smear is perhaps the most common procedure used.

After the smear is prepared and air dried, it is usually stained with Wright's stain. Its use is primarily for white blood cell differentials and morphologic studies. Because the spun smear is an automated method and not that commonly used a procedure, only the coverslip and slide wedge methods will be discussed.

THE COVERSLIP PROCEDURE

1. If blood from a fingerstick is to be used, wipe away the first drop and use the second. If venous blood is to be used, a drop of blood 1 to 2 mm in diameter from the needle of the syringe or evacuated system will suffice. In both cases, the drop of blood must be placed in the center of the coverslip.

2. Use 22 × 22-mm coverslips. The coverslips must be made of glass, not plastic, and they *must be scrupulously clean.* If there is any doubt, first soak them in 70% ethyl alcohol and then wipe dry with lint-free 4 × 4-inch gauze before using.

3. Holding the coverslip (onto which the drop of blood has been placed) between the thumb and forefinger by adjacent corners, place a second coverslip immediately and gently over the first so that it resembles Figure 13-1.

4. The second coverslip should be held at adjacent corners similarly to the first. As soon as they come together, the blood will spread.

5. Just before the blood is completely spread, take hold of the free corners and rapidly pull them apart in an even, horizontal, lateral pull as indicated in Figure 13-2.

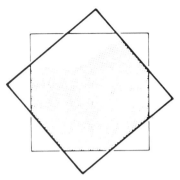

Fig. 13-1. Position of coverslips when making a coverslip blood smear. (From Brown, B. A.: Hematology: Principles and Procedures, 4th Ed. Philadelphia, Lea & Febiger, 1984.)

6. Let them air dry. *Do not blow on them.*
7. The coverslips are now ready for staining.

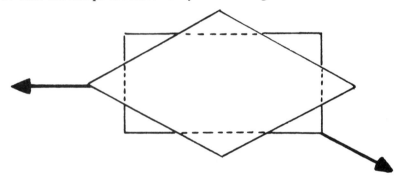

Fig. 13-2. Directions coverslips should be pulled when making a coverslip blood smear.

THE SLIDE WEDGE PROCEDURE

1. Glass slides, 1 × 3 inches (25 × 75 mm), are used to make the slide wedge smear. The slides, like the coverslips, *must be scrupulously clean.* Questionably clean slides should first be soaked in 70% ethyl alcohol and then wiped dry with a lint-free 4 × 4-inch gauze.

2. In the preparation of the slide wedge smear, a spreader must be used. It may be a 1 × 3-inch glass slide with the corners of one end cut off (see Figure 13-3), a hemocytometer coverslip, or simply another 1 × 3-inch glass slide with no alterations. The latter is the most commonly used spreader.

3. If blood from a fingerstick is used, wipe away the first drop and use the second. Venous blood may be applied directly from the syringe or evacuated system needle. Blood may also be applied from the evacuated system by holding two applicator sticks close together and dipping them into the well-mixed EDTA tube.

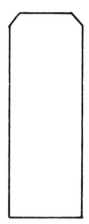

Fig. 13-3. A 1 × 3-inch glass slide with corners altered for use as a spreader.

4. The drop of blood should be no more than 1 to 2 mm in diameter. Place the drop in the middle of the slide toward the frosted end. It should be approximately 1 cm in front of the frosted portion. *Make the smear immediately after you have applied the drop of blood.*

5. Place the slide on a flat surface and hold securely. Use the thumb and index finger of the other hand to hold the spreader.

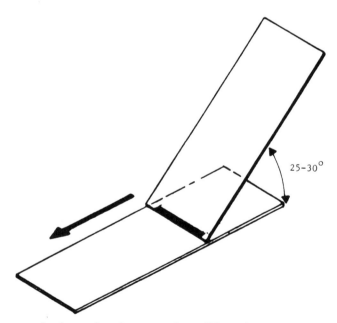

Fig. 13-4. Proper angle of spreader when preparing a slide wedge smear. (From Bauer, J. D.: Clinical Laboratory Methods, 9th Ed. St. Louis, C. V. Mosby, 1982.)

6. Place the end of the spreader just in front of the drop of blood at an angle of 25 to 30° (see Figure 13-4).

7. Now draw the spreader back toward the drop of blood. Allow the blood to spread in the angle between the slide and the spreader. If an unaltered glass slide is used as the spreader, just before the blood has spread to the edges, push the spreader ahead of the drop of blood.

8. Push the spreader the entire length of the slide. Make sure that you hold the spreader firmly against the other slide, and that you make the smear in one smooth movement. Avoid any jerky movements.

9. Air dry as quickly as possible to prevent distortion of the red blood cells. This may be accomplished by rapidly waving the slides back and forth in the air. Be sure to prepare two smears.

10. The smears are now ready for staining.

11. A well-prepared blood smear has a thick portion beginning at the point of application which is drawn out into a feathery edge (see Figure 13-5).

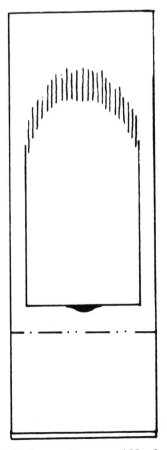

Fig. 13-5. Diagrammatic sketch of properly prepared blood smear.

Note:
Two main conditions affect the viscosity of the blood. Polycythemia (hemoglobin of 18 g/dl or greater) will increase the viscosity of the blood. Anemia (hemoglobin of 7 g/dl or less) will cause a decrease in the viscosity. When the viscosity is increased, a thinner slide is needed. To accomplish this, decrease the angle between the spreader and the slide. When the viscosity is abnormally low, a thicker slide is in order. To make thicker slides, increase the angle between the spreader and the slides.

BIBLIOGRAPHY

1. Bauer, J. D.: Clinical Laboratory Methods, 9th Ed. St. Louis, C. V. Mosby, 1982.
2. Brown, B. A.: Hematology: Principles and Procedures, 5th Ed. Philadelphia, Lea & Febiger, 1988.

Chapter 14

GENERAL PROCEDURE FOR THE UNOPETTE Brand HEMATOLOGY SYSTEM

The UNOPETTE is a microcollection system developed by Becton Dickinson. Basically, it consists of a reservoir and a capillary pipette that is self-filling and self-measuring. The system has been developed for manual use and for use with automated equipment. Individual UNOPETTE systems are available to do white blood cell counts, red blood cell counts, platelet counts, hemoglobins, eosinophil counts, erythrocyte fragility, reticulocyte staining, sodium and potassium determinations, and for use on the Coulter counter. Procedural variations exist between the systems, but except for the reticulocyte determination, the patient-sample collecting steps are basically similar. The UNOPETTE manual white blood cell count is described in the following section to illustrate the sample collection steps.

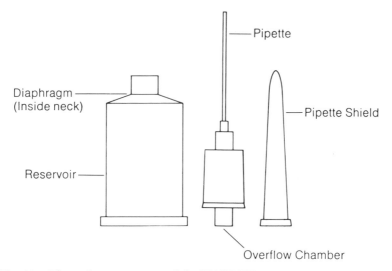

Fig. 14-1. The major components of the UNOPETTE system.

1. Place the reservoir on a flat surface, holding it securely with one hand. Using the other hand, firmly push the tip of the pipette shield through the diaphragm in the neck of the reservoir and then remove the pipette shield.

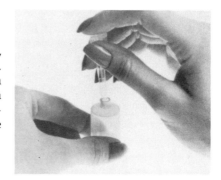

Fig. 14-2.

2. Next, remove the pipette shield from around the pipette by a simple twist.

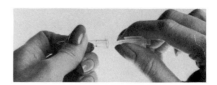

Fig. 14-3.

3. Hold the pipette almost horizontal while touching the tip of the pipette to the patient's blood. The pipette will fill by capillary action. The filling is complete and will stop automatically when the blood reaches the end of the capillary bore in the neck of the pipette.

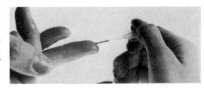

4. Wipe any excess blood from the outside of the capillary pipette, making sure that none of the sample has accidentally been removed from the bore of the pipette.

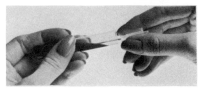

5. Next, squeeze the reservoir slightly to remove some of the air without expelling any of the liquid. Maintain this slight pressure on the reservoir.

Fig. 14-4.

6. Covering the overflow chamber of the pipette with the index finger, place the pipette securely into the neck of the reservoir.

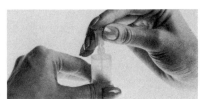

7. Release the pressure on the reservoir and remove the index finger from the pipette. The negative pressure will draw the blood into the diluent.

Fig. 14-5.

8. Squeeze the reservoir *gently* two to three times to rinse the capillary bore. Force the diluent up into, *but not out of,* the overflow chamber of the pipette. Release the pressure each time to return the mixture to the reservoir.

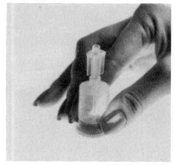

Fig. 14-6.

9. Now place the index finger over the upper opening (the inserted pipette) and gently invert the system several times to thoroughly mix the blood and the diluent.

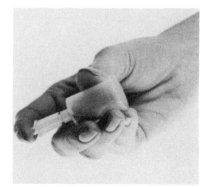

Fig. 14-7.

10. Convert to a dropper assembly by withdrawing the pipette from the reservoir and reseating it securely in the reverse position.

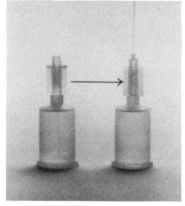

Fig. 14-8.

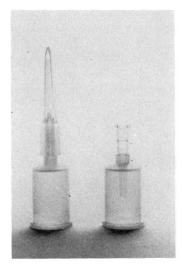

11. For transporting and temporary storage, place the capillary shield loosely over the exposed pipette.

Fig. 14-9.

BIBLIOGRAPHY

1. Laboratory Procedure Using the UNOPETTE Brand System. Rutherford, NJ, Becton Dickinson, 1977.

Chapter **15**

SPECIAL COLLECTION TECHNIQUES

Most laboratory procedures in which blood is used require only a routine venipuncture. The sample must simply be collected in the correct tube. For some tests, if the specimens cannot be assayed immediately, there are additional requirements, such as that the specimen should be refrigerated, frozen, or protected from the light. Several of the tests in the second group, and their specific demands, are listed in Chapter 16, General Collection Requirements.

A few laboratory tests require distinctly special manipulations in addition to the venipuncture, such as prewarming the collection tube or administering a solution to the patient. Still other tests have nothing to do with venipunctures but are, nevertheless, invasive techniques, utilizing one or more specific manipulations.

This section does not attempt to discuss every laboratory test that requires special collection techniques. Its scope is limited to those tests most often encountered in a general care hospital or other health care facility.

CROSSMATCHES

Purpose

When obtaining a blood sample from any patient, the greatest care must be exercised to make sure that the sample is taken from the correct patient and that the sample tubes are properly labeled. This statement cannot be made often and emphatically enough. *Nowhere is the above statement more important, however, than when obtaining a blood sample from a patient who may possibly need a blood transfusion.*

Ordering procedures vary from hospital to hospital. Generally, however, a *type and Rh* are ordered on all pregnant females. This may be known as a "prenatal screen." The blood is typed to see whether it is type O, A, B, or AB and to see whether it is either Rh-positive or Rh-negative.

Surgeons will often order a *type and screen* on their patients. The patients may or may not need blood transfusions. This depends on the amount of blood loss during the operation. The type and screen includes the type and Rh determinations, and the patient's blood is tested for the presence of specific antibodies. If the patient does have an antibody, and if during surgery a transfusion is required, the laboratory will have had time to acquire compatible blood and have it on hand.

At present, blood is *usually* crossmatched before it is transfused. The word usually is used because there are situations, such as severe hemorrhaging, in which any blood is better than no blood, and the time required for a crossmatch makes it an impractical procedure.

Basically, the crossmatch includes the ABO-type and Rh-factor determinations, a screen of the recipient's blood for specific antibodies, and tests to see whether the recipient's serum has antibodies that will react against the newly infused donor's red blood cells—in other words, a check to see whether the donor's blood and the recipient's blood are compatible. Infusion of incompatible blood can cause clumping (agglutination) or rupturing (lysis) of the red blood cells in the recipient's circulatory system.

Phlebotomy Procedure

1. *Make sure of the patient's identity.* Do not ask, "Are you Mr. Smith?" Ask the patient to give you his full name. Next, check the patient's hospital identification arm band against the name on the requisition form. If the patient is unconscious or otherwise incoherent, *have a nurse positively identify the patient.*
2. Draw at least one red-top tube (without polymer gel), two if possible. Label the tubes with the following information:
   a. patient's name
   b. date and time the specimen was collected
   c. patient's hospital number
   d. initials of the person doing the venipuncture
   e. the birthday of the patient may also be required
3. Make sure to collect the blood specimen carefully so that hemolysis of the red blood cells does not occur.
4. Most hospitals have some type of identification band that is placed on the patient's wrist as soon as the specimen has been collected. The bands are usually made of soft plastic, and after they have been attached, must be cut to be removed.
5. In most hospitals there is also a label that has a preprinted identification number identical to the one on the wrist band. This label must be affixed to the tube of blood. This same identification number will be placed on the unit of blood that has been crossmatched. In addition to the patient's name and other information, the nurse, before infusing the blood, will check to see whether the identification number on the patient's wrist band corresponds with the identification number on the unit of blood.

Warning:
When obtaining a blood sample where there is a possibility that blood

may be transfused, *check and double check.* A unit of blood given to the wrong person could kill, and lawsuits for negligence are not fun.

Purpose

The detection of septicemia.

Preparation of the Patient

1. Explain to the patient, if he is coherent, that the physician has ordered a series of tests and you will have to stick him several times.
2. Using an alcohol swab, clean the arm(s), making concentric rings from the inside out.
3. Perform the above procedure again, this time using an iodine swab.
4. Let the iodine dry before doing the venipuncture. Once the iodine has been applied, *do not "feel" for the vein again unless you have "sterilized" your own fingers as you did the venipuncture site.*

Phlebotomy Procedure

Note:
Each microbiology laboratory uses its own particular blood culture system. The protocol for the collection of blood cultures also differs from hospital to hospital. Nevertheless, certain procedural steps are common to all blood culture methods.

1. Paint the septum of the blood culture bottle(s) with iodine.
2. For the first or primary blood culture, if possible, collect a blood sample from each arm. The amount of blood to be drawn depends on the blood culture system used. Draw the sample only in sterile syringes.
3. After withdrawing the blood, replace the needle used to make the venipuncture with a new sterile one. Inject the sample into the blood culture bottle and quickly, but gently, mix to avoid clotting.
4. In subsequent blood cultures, one venipuncture will be enough; however, each one should be obtained from alternate arms. Also, the amount of blood required will depend on whether the laboratory uses a one- or two-bottle system for the recovery of aerobic and anaerobic organisms (see Figure 15-1).
Important:
Label each bottle with the patient's name, the date, time the culture was taken, and the arm from which the blood was drawn.

5. When returning to the laboratory, you may be required to "vent" one of the blood culture bottles if a two-bottle system is used. Check with the laboratory regarding the proper protocol for this procedure.
Note:
In some hospitals, if the patient is placed on antibiotic therapy before

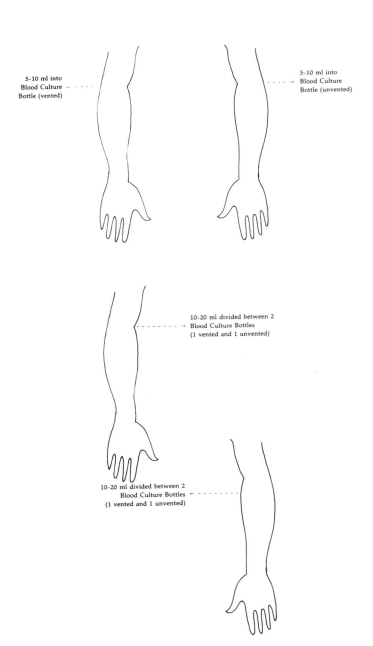

Fig. 15-1. Protocol for the collection of blood cultures.

the blood culture is taken, the blood sample is placed in an "antimicrobial removing device" before being inoculated into blood culture bottles. There is no difference in the phlebotomy procedure. Some of these devices contain a membrane that you must be careful not to puncture.

Values

Normal blood cultures should be sterile. The growth of microorganisms in the blood is a life-threatening situation.

ORAL GLUCOSE TOLERANCE TEST (GTT)

Purpose

1. To confirm diabetes mellitus.
2. To aid in the diagnosis of hypoglycemia and malabsorption syndrome.

Preparation of Patient

1. The patient must not eat, smoke, drink coffee or alcohol, or exercise strenuously for at least 10 hours before or during the test.
2. If the GTT is to be done on an outpatient, schedule the time the patient should arrive at the laboratory, explain how many blood samples will be required, and encourage the patient to bring something to read since the procedure will take some time to complete.

Phlebotomy Procedure

1. Obtain the patient's height and weight. Using these figures, calculate the amount of glucose solution to give the patient. A number of calculators are available to use for this purpose. An example of one such calculator is illustrated in Figure 15-2.
2. Draw a fasting sample. It should be collected in a gray-top tube. A fasting urine specimen should also be collected at the same time.
3. Give the patient the predetermined amount of glucose solution to drink. *Note the time.* Make sure the glucose solution is chilled. Instruct the patient to drink all the solution. This should be done within a 5-minute time limit. *Make sure you watch the patient drink the glucose solution.*
   Note:
   Some institutions determine the glucose level of the fasting sample before administering the glucose solution. If the fasting glucose is high, the physician is contacted for instructions before the test is continued.

4. Draw a specimen at 30 minutes, 1 hour, 2 hours, and 3 hours (or more if required) after you have given the patient the glucose solution to drink. Also, collect a urine specimen each time you stick the patient. Note the time each blood and urine sample was collected.

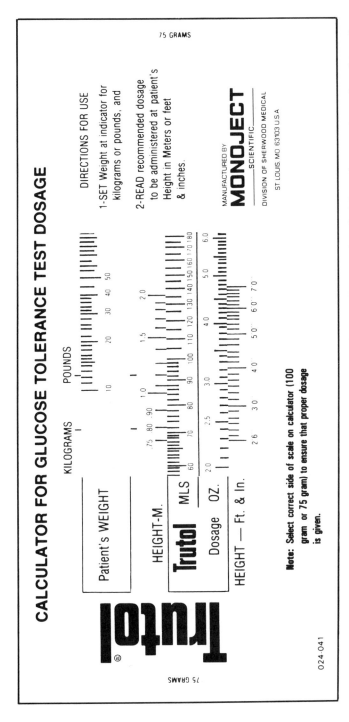

Fig. 15-2. Example of a calculator used to determine the amount of glucose solution to be administered to a patient when doing the glucose tolerance test.

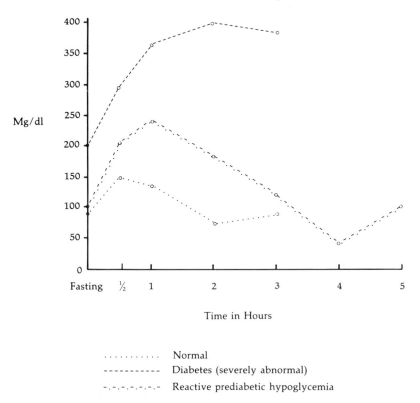

Mg/dl

Time in Hours

. . . . Normal
- - - - - - - - - - Diabetes (severely abnormal)
-.-.-.-.-.-.- Reactive prediabetic hypoglycemia

Fig. 15-3. Glucose tolerance curve.

Note:
If, at any time during the test, the patient feels either faint or nauseated, have him lie down. It would be advisable to have an emesis basin and towel readily available just in case the patient needs to vomit. If vomiting occurs within the first half-hour of the test, discontinue, notify the physician, and if appropriate, reschedule for another day. On the other hand, if vomiting occurs approximately 1¼ hours after the test has started, have the patient lie down and complete the test. If, after repeated attempts to do the oral GTT, the patient continues to vomit within the first half-hour, the IV GTT may have to be considered. Encourage the patient to drink water throughout the test to promote adequate urine excretion. If the patient should develop severe hypoglycemia, take a blood sample, note the time, and alert a physician. Discontinue the test.
Warning:
The glucose tolerance test is a "timed" test. Most patients on whom a GTT is being done are borderline diabetics. As can be noted from the graph in Figure 15-3, in order for the physician to make a correct diagno-

sis, it is important that each specimen be drawn as close to the correct time as possible. *If, for any reason, you are unable to collect a specimen at the appointed time, alert the appropriate laboratory supervisor immediately.*

COLD AGGLUTININS

Purpose

1. To help confirm primary atypical pneumonia caused by *Mycoplasma pneumoniae.*
2. To provide additional diagnostic evidence for some viral infections (e.g., Epstein-Barr virus and cytomegalovirus) and disorders caused by lymphomas.

Phlebotomy Procedure

1. Collect the sample in a red-top tube. Approximately 30 minutes before sticking the patient, place the tube in a 37°C incubator to prewarm. In order to keep the tube as warm as possible, carry the tube in your palm when going to the patient's room.
2. After collecting the specimen, bring the tube back to the laboratory as soon as possible. Again, carry the tube in your palm. When you get to the laboratory, place the specimen into a 37°C incubator or water bath. Alert the serology laboratory immediately.

   Note:

   Prevent hemolysis when collecting the sample. Also, if you allow the specimen to get cold, the "cold agglutinins" will coat the red blood cells and leave none in the serum for testing.

Values

Normally, titers for cold agglutinins are 1:16 or less.

FIBRIN DEGRADATION PRODUCTS

From the basic coagulation scheme, you should remember that thrombin induces clot formation by the conversion of fibrinogen to fibrin. If the process stopped there, all of us at some time would find our circulation impaired because we would be full of clots. But once a wound has healed, the clot is removed by the process of fibrinolysis. A substance known as plasmin digests fibrin (the clot), generating fibrin degradation products (FDP) called X, Y, D, and E. These degradation products have an anticoagulant action.

Sometimes a pathologic state occurs in which generalized clotting takes place in the small blood vessels. In fact, the clotting may be localized to one or a few organs. This phenomenon may be caused by infectious agents, solid-tumor malignancies, leukemia, or hemolytic disorders, to name just a few of the diseases. This complex entity is known as disseminated intravascular coagulation (DIC).

Disseminated intravascular coagulation is a paradox in that clotting occurs that causes bleeding. In other words, an excess of thrombin exists that causes enhanced clotting. This enhanced clotting stimulates excessive fibrinolysis (with its degradation products) and allows bleeding.

When DIC is suspected, the platelet count and fibrinogen determination, the two most important tests, are the minimum needed. The primary test for DIC involves detection of fibrin degradation products.

Purpose

The detection of fibrin degradation products, which aids in confirming the diagnosis of disseminated intravascular coagulation.

Phlebotomy Procedure

1. Because DIC is a life-threatening condition, an early and accurate diagnosis is essential. Extreme care must be taken to avoid hemolysis of the specimens during collection.

2. Since a platelet count and a fibrinogen level will be ordered, it will be necessary to collect specimens in both a blue-top tube and a purple-top tube. In addition, a red-top tube specimen should be carefully collected in order that possible hemolysis can be observed.

3. A commercial test, the Thrombo-Wellcotest, is used in most laboratories to detect the presence of FDP. The specimen to be used for this test must be collected in special glass tubes containing an enzyme inhibitor and thrombin. The specimen may be 2 ml of either whole blood or urine.

BLEEDING TIME

Purpose

To detect platelet function disorders.

Preparation of the Patient

1. Explain to the patient that a bleeding time is a test to see how long it will take for the patient's blood to stop bleeding and to form a clot.

2. Unless the patient is an infant, outline to the patient how the test will be done. Explain that the test will take approximately 10 to 20 minutes to complete.

3. Let the patient know that he may experience some discomfort from the incision and the cuff of the sphygmomanometer (if one is used).

4. Sometimes, the test is less traumatic and the time passes faster for children if their assistance is solicited in watching the stopwatch and letting the laboratorian know when to blot the blood.

Phlebotomy Procedure

1. Ivy commercial method

a. The arm must be in a supine position on a steady support, with the volar surface exposed.
b. The incision is best performed 5 cm below and parallel to the antecubital crease. Avoid surface veins.

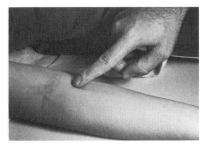

Fig. 15-4.

c. Clean the area with 70% ethyl alcohol. If the arm is very hairy, lightly shave the area.

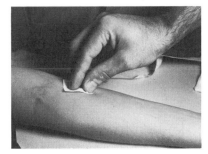

Fig. 15-5.

d. Remove the incision-making instrument from its package. Be careful not to contaminate the instrument by touching or resting the blade-slot end on any unsterile surface. Ready it for use by removing any safety devices.

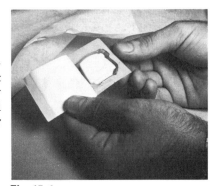

Fig. 15-6.

e. Place a sphygmomanometer cuff on the upper arm and inflate to 40 mm Hg. Monitor the sphygmomanometer frequently to make sure the pressure remains at 40 mm Hg throughout the test.

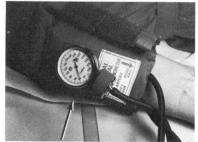

Fig. 15-7.

f. The test should be started within 60 seconds after the blood pressure cuff has been inflated. Place the incision-making instrument firmly on the fore-arm, but do not press. A horizontal incision is the most sensitive technique for the bleeding time test. Depress the trigger and start the stopwatch simultaneously. Remove the incision-making instrument almost immediately after depressing the trigger.

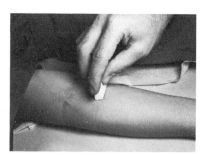

Fig. 15-8.

g. Blot the flow of blood every 30 seconds. Place the filter paper close to the incision, but do not touch the edge of the wound because this may disturb the platelet plug.

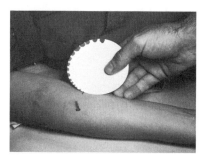

Fig. 15-9.

h. Continue to blot every 30 seconds until the blood no longer stains the filter paper. Stop the stopwatch and note the time to the nearest 30 seconds.

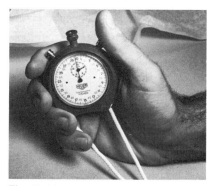

Fig. 15-10.

i. Remove the sphygmomanometer cuff. Gently clean the arm with an antiseptic swab and place a butterfly bandage across the incision. The patient should keep the bandage in place for at least 24 hours.

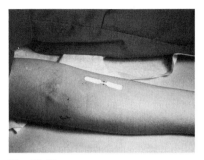

Fig. 15-11.

Values

Time ranges will vary depending on the brand of instrument used. Published reports indicate a mean bleeding time in normal patients to be 5.4, 5.7, and 4.5 minutes, respectively, for the Hemalet, Simplate, and Surgicutt devices.

2. Duke method
   a. Clean either an earlobe or finger with 70% alcohol.
   b. Using a sterile long-point blood lancet, make a puncture and, at the same time, start the stopwatch.
   c. Blot the blood with filter paper every 30 seconds. Avoid touching the wound in order not to disturb the platelet clot.
   d. When the blood no longer stains the filter paper, stop the timer. Record the time to the nearest 30 seconds.
   Values: 1 to 3 minutes, with 3 to 6 minutes being borderline.

HEPARIN LOCK PROCEDURE

In certain situations, multiple draws must be made either in a short period of time (e.g., checking electrolytes) or as timed samples (e.g., the glucose or insulin tolerance test) on patients with veins that are next to impossible to locate, much less stick. This situation often occurs with debilitated patients, usually in the Intensive and Cardiac Care Units, or with extremely obese patients. In these situations, it may be appropriate to use a heparin lock. This allows the laboratory to obtain the required number of samples with minimum discomfort, not to speak of psychologic trauma, to the patient. Regulations differ from hospital to hospital, but *since heparin is a drug, the physician's permission will be required to insert this device.* Also, this procedure is somewhat tedious and demands special precautions. *Only approved individuals should attempt to insert and use the heparin lock.*

Equipment

1. 21-gauge butterfly with heparin lock
2. heparin lock flush solution, 19 USP per ml
3. TUBEX hypodermic syringe
4. gauze

5. paper tape
6. tuberculin syringes
7. 5-ml syringes with 21-gauge needles
8. IV support board

Phlebotomy Procedure

1. Using green soap and iodine, surgically clean the area where the heparin lock is to be inserted.
2. Vent the heparin lock with a 21-gauge needle.
3. Insert the butterfly into the vein and let the blood flow freely into the tubing and out the 21-gauge needle. Make sure that no air remains in the system.
4. Now connect a 5-ml syringe to the 21-gauge needle and obtain the first blood sample.
5. Remove the syringe and the 21-gauge needle. Using a TUBEX hypodermic syringe, flush the heparin lock with 1.0 ml of the 10 U heparin solution.
6. Now place the patient's arm on an IV support board and secure the heparin lock, using gauze and paper tape.
7. To obtain subsequent samples
   a. Clean the surface of the heparin lock with 70% alcohol.
   b. Insert a tuberculin syringe with a 25-gauge needle and slowly withdraw 1.0 ml of heparin-blood mixture. Discard.
   c. Quickly insert into the heparin lock a 21-gauge needle with a 5-ml syringe. Slowly aspirate the desired amount of blood sample.
   d. Remove the syringe and 21-gauge needle. Again flush the heparin lock with 1.0 ml of the 10 U heparin solution as previously described.
   e. Repeat steps 7a through d, as necessary.

BIBLIOGRAPHY

1. Barber, J.: Basic coagulation. Lab. Med., *9:*40, 1978.
2. Bartlett, R. C., Ellner, P. D., and Washington, J. A., II: Blood Cultures, Cumitech 1, Washington, D.C., American Society for Microbiology, 1974.
3. Bauer, J. D.: Clinical Laboratory Methods, 9th Ed. St. Louis, C. V. Mosby, 1982.
4. Brown, B. A.: Hematology: Principles and Procedures, 5th Ed. Philadelphia, Lea & Febiger, 1988.
5. Burns, E. R.: The Hemalet bleeding time device. Lab. Med., *17:*745, 1986.
6. DaCunha, J. P., Ford, R. D., and Glover, S. M. (eds.): Diagnostics. Springfield, PA, Intermed Communications, Inc., 1981.
7. Gralnick, H. R.: Intravascular Coagulation 1. Differential diagnosis and conditioning mechanisms. Postgrad. Med., *62:*68, 1977.
8. McKenzie, S. B.: Textbook of Hematology. Philadelphia, Lea & Febiger, 1988.
9. Patel, K.: Heparin lock procedure. Personal Communication, 1983.
10. Reynolds, J. B.: Detection of Fibrinogen/Fibrin Degradation (Split) Products fdp/fsp. Research Park, NC, Burroughs Wellcome Co., 1981.
11. Smith, C.: Surgicutt: A device for modified template bleeding times. J. Med. Tech., *3:*229, 1986.

CHAPTER 16

GENERAL COLLECTION REQUIREMENTS

Below is an illustrative list of chemical, hematologic, and serologic tests done in many laboratories. In large laboratories many more tests are performed than those listed below, whereas small laboratories may do very few in the list. Good phlebotomy technique includes more than just collecting a specimen in the proper evacuated tube. **It is important that attention be paid to any special instructions required by the testing laboratory.**

CODE

B—Light blue-top evacuated tube
Gr—Gray-top evacuated tube
Gn—Green-top evacuated tube
L—Lavender-top evacuated tube
NB—Navy blue–top evacuated tube
R—Red-top evacuated tube
S—Use syringe

Test	Code	Special Instructions
ABO type	R	At least 7.0 ml clot
Acid phosphatase (PAP)	R	Freeze if not delivered to lab in 4 hours
Albumin	R	
Alcohol	L or Gr	
Alkaline phosphatase	R	
Amylase	R	
Antinuclear antibodies (ANA)	R	Avoid lipemic or hemolyzed serum
B-12, vitamin	R	Avoid hemolysis and protect from light
Bilirubin, total or direct	R	Protect from light

Test	Code	Special Instructions
Blood urea nitrogen (BUN)	R	
Calcium	R	
Carcinoembryonic antigen (CEA)	R or L	
Cardiac enzymes	R	
CBC	L	
Cholesterol, HDL	R	Collect after 8- to 12-hour fast
Cholesterol, total	R	
Clot retraction	S	Place 3 ml in 13 × 100-mm test tube; place in 37°C water bath and allow to clot
Cold agglutinins	R	Incubate blood at 37°C until clotted; separate immediately after blood clots
Complement, C3	R	
Complement, C4	R	Freeze serum
Complement, total (CH50)	R	Let clot in refrigerator; separate immediately and freeze serum
Complement, total (CH100)	R	Let clot in refrigerator; separate immediaely and freeze serum
Cortisol	R or L	
CPK isoenzymes	R	
C-reactive protein (CRP)	R	
Creatinine	R	
Creatinine phosphokinase (CPK), total	R	
Digitoxin	R	
Digoxin	R	
Dilantin	R	
Electrolytes (Na, K, Cl, CO)	R	Avoid hemolysis
Febrile agglutination	R	
Ferritin	R	
Fibrinogen	B	Maximum draw
Folate, serum	R	Avoid hemolysis
Fungal serologies	R	
Gamma-glutamyl transpepsidase (GGT)	R	
Gentamicin	R	Label peak or trough
Glucose, fasting	R	
Glucose, 2-hour postprandial	R	

Test	Code	Special Instructions
Glucose tolerance	R	3-hour: 5 specimens 5-hour: 7 specimens (urine sample for each interval)
Glycosylated hemoglobin	L	
Hematocrit	L	
Hemoglobin	L	
Hemoglobin electrophoresis	L	
Hepatitis profiles	R	
Beta-human chorionic gonadotropin (HCG)	R	
Human immunodeficiency virus (HIV)	R	
Human leukocyte antigen (HLA-B27)	R and Gn	Gn-donor, R-recipient; do not freeze or refrigerate; record date and time collected
Iron, serum	R	Avoid hemolysis
Lactic dehydrogenase (LDH)	R	
LDH isoenzymes	R	
Lead	L	
Lipase	R	
Lithium	R	
Liver profile	R	
Magnesium	R	Avoid hemolysis
Mononucleosis serology	R	
Osmolality, serum	R	
Partial thromboplastin time (PTT)	B	Maximum draw
Phenobarbitol	R	
Phosphorus	R	
Platelet count	L	
Potassium	R	Avoid hemolysis
Procainamide	R	
Prostate specific antigen (PSA)	R	Freeze specimen if not delivered to lab within 4 hours
Prostatic acid phosphatase (PAP)	R	Freeze specimen if not delivered to lab within 4 hours
Prothrombin time (PT)	B	Maximum draw
Quinidine	R	
Rapid plasma reagin (RPR)	R or L	
Reticulocyte count	L	
Rheumatoid arthritis serology (RA)	R	
Rubella titer	R	
Salicylates	R	

Test	Code	Special Instructions
Sedimentation rate	L	
SGOT (AST)	R	
SGPT (ALT)	R	
SMA-profiles	R	
Sodium	R	
Streptozyme	R	
T, T	R	
T4/T8 ratio	L and Gn	Blood smear needed; do not freeze or refrigerate
Theophylline	R	
Thioridazine (Mellaril)	R	Protect from light
Thyroid antibodies	R	
Thyroid profiles	R	
Thyroid-stimulating hormones (TSH)	R	
Thyroxine-binding globulin (TBG)	R	
Tobramycin	R	Label peak or trough
Total iron-binding capacity (TIBC)	R	
Transferrin	R	
Triglycerides	R	
Uric acid	R	
Viral serologies	R	
Western blot	R	
Zinc	NB	

BIBLIOGRAPHY

1. Compendium of Services. Valdosta, GA, Doctors Laboratory, Inc., 1990.
2. Jacobs, D. S., Kasten, B. L., Jr., DeMott, W. R., and Wolfson, W. L. (eds.): Laboratory Test Handbook, 2nd Ed. Baltimore, Williams & Wilkins, 1990.
3. Kaplan, A., Szabo, L. L., and Opheim, K. E.: Clinical Chemistry: Interpretation and Technique, 3rd Ed. Philadelphia, Lea & Febiger, 1988.
4. Tietz, N. W. (ed.): Fundamentals of Clinical Chemistry, 2nd Ed. Philadelphia, W. B. Saunders, 1988.

APPENDIX

Sources for Educational Material

Below is a limited list of sources for educational materials that are suitable for both primary and continuing education in phlebotomy. In addition, most of the distributors of phlebotomy supplies will graciously send printed or video materials regarding their products for distribution or display.

1. *Becton Dickinson VACUTAINER Systems*
   Rutherford, New Jersey 07070-1598
   Telephone: (800) 631-0174

   Becton Dickinson has for purchase a very good videotape entitled *Be Kind to Tiny Feet.* It shows how to do capillary punctures on the heels of infants and discusses the importance of limiting the depth of heel punctures to 2.4 mm. Other materials are available including several excellent wall charts dealing with trouble shooting, technique, and coding and laboratory use for their evacuated tubes.

2. *Educational Materials for Health Professionals, Inc.*
   607 Watervliet Avenue
   Dayton, Ohio 45420
   Telephone: (513) 254-0990

   This organization has several instructional units that are suitable for phlebotomists. Three videotapes covering capillary puncture, venipuncture, and the making of a blood film are available. Self-instructional booklets can be purchased separately to complement the videotapes. These booklets contain learning exercises and self-evaluation questions. The videotapes were made in 1986 prior to universal precautions. Overlooking this drawback, they nevertheless do a good job of demonstrating proper techniques. Prepared in 1990 and available in booklet form only is a self-instructional packet on laboratory safety.

3. *American Society of Clinical Pathologists*
   2100 West Harrison Street
   Chicago, Illinois 60612-3798
   Telephone: (800) 621-4142

   The ASCP has produced four excellent videotapes. *Blood Collection: The Pediatric Patient* provides information about performing heelsticks, fingersticks, and venipunctures using a butterfly needle. *Blood Collection: The Routine Venipuncture* demonstrates the routine venipuncture based on

NCCLS and OSHA standards. *Laboratory Safety and Infection Control* covers the major risks associated with the clinical laboratory and precautions to be taken. *Blood Collection: Special Procedures* covers blood cultures, type and cross-match, special transport, cold agglutinins, the modified Ivy bleeding time, therapeutic drug monitoring, and glucose tolerance testing. Details that are discussed for each procedure include site selection and preparation, patient identification, equipment used, and procedure and quality assurance considerations.

4. *Division of Continuing Education*
   Medical College of Georgia
   Augusta, Georgia 30912-1400

The *Learning Laboratorian Series* is published quarterly and may be purchased by a yearly subscription or by the volume of your choice. In addition to a clear explanation of the subject, each volume includes learning objectives, a key word list that defines the meaning and usage of terms that may be unfamiliar, and a self-assessment examination. Continuing education credit may be obtained. Three of the volumes of interest to phlebotomists are *Phlebotomy, Infectious Diseases,* and *Laboratory Safety*.

5. *AHC/MLO AIDS Education Kit*
   67 Peachtree Park Drive
   Atlanta, Georgia 30309
   Telephone: (800) 554-1032 In Georgia: *(404) 262-7436*

Using NCCLS guidelines, universal precautions as recommended by CDC, and proposed OSHA regulations, Medical Laboratory Observer has developed the videotape *Laboratory Safety: Containing HIV and HBV—Barriers for Your Protection*. The video shows how transmission and infection can occur and what protective measures individuals who work in the clinical laboratory should take. This video is a very good one for phlebotomists, particularly if they are also involved in specimen preparation.

6. *Elektro Assemblies, Inc.*
   522 N.W. Sixth Avenue
   Rochester, Minnesota 55901
   Telephone: (800) 533-1558

Elektro Assemblies, Inc., manufactures an inexpensive phlebotomy training device called the *Veni-Dot*. The simulation to an actual arm and veins is excellent. It is portable, easy to assemble, simple to use, and easily stored.

Phlebotomy Certifying Agencies

1. *American Society of Clinical Pathologists (ASCP)*
Board of Registry
P.O. Box 12270
Chicago, Illinois 60612
Telephone: (312) 738-1336

Frequency of examination:	Once per year. Given only in designated cities.
Examination format:	Multiple choice.
Eligibility routes:	a) High school diploma or equivalent and completion of a NAACLS approved program within the last 5 years.
	OR
	b) High school diploma or equivalent and completion of an acceptable formal program.
	OR
	c) High school diploma or equivalent and 1 year of full-time work experience in phlebotomy within the last 5 years.
Certification:	PBT(ASCP)
Recertification:	Once certified, recertification is not required.

2. *American Society of Phlebotomy Technicians (ASPT)*
P.O. Box 1831
Hickory, North Carolina 28603
Telephone: (704) 322-1334

Frequency of examination:	On demand. If approved, may be given at the candidate's place of employment or training.
Examination format:	Multiple choice and practical.
Eligibility routes:	a) At least 6 months of full-time work experience in phlebotomy.
	OR
	b) One year of part-time work experience in phlebotomy.
	OR
	c) Completion of a training program that has been reviewed by ASPT.
Certification:	CPT(ASPT)
Recertification:	Certification must be renewed yearly by either reexamination or 6 contact hours per year of medically related continuing education

3. *National Certification Agency for Medical Laboratory Personnel (NCA)*
   2021 L Street NW, Suite 400
   Washington, D.C. 20036
   Telephone: (202) 857-1023

Frequency of examination:	Twice per year. Given only in designated cities.
Examination format:	Multiple choice.
Eligibility routes:	a) Completion of a formal education program.
	OR
	b) One year of full-time work experience in phlebotomy.
Certification:	CLPlb(NCA)
Recertification:	Recertification is every 2 years by 20 contact hours of continuing education or every 4 years by reexamination.

4. *National Phlebotomy Association (NPA)*
   2623 Bladenburg Road, N.E.
   Washington, D.C. 20018
   Telephone: (202) 636-4515

Frequency of examination:	Varies with need. The NPA has a Reclamation Clause wherein experienced phlebotomists may be certified without examination.
Examination format:	Written portion and practical portion.
Eligibility routes:	a) Working phlebotomist with 1 year of work experience in phlebotomy.
	OR
	b) Completion of an NPA-approved training program.
	OR
	c) Fifty-four contact hours of phlebotomy education if candidate has less than 1 year of work experience in phlebotomy.
Certification:	CPT(NPA)
Recertification:	Recertification yearly by 18 contact hours of continuing education credits.

INDEX

Page numbers in italics refer to figures.

Abbreviations, for laboratory tests, 35-37
  medical, meanings of, 31-35
Acci-Guard, *67*, 68
Acquired immunodeficiency syndrome
  (AIDS), 10, 13, 14, 15, 67
Activated partial thromboplastin time (APTT),
  50
Agglutinin(s), cold. *See* Cold agglutinin(s)
Aggregating agent(s), 48
AIDS. *See* Acquired immunodeficiency syn-
  drome (AIDS)
Airborne transmission, of infectious disease
  agents, 13
American Society for Medical Techology, code
  of ethics, 8
American Society of Clinical Pathologists
  (ASCP), 4, 121
American Society of Phlebotomy Technicians
  (ASPT), 4, 121
Anemia, 96
Anticoagulant(s), 38, 62, 64
Aorta, 47, *47*
Aortic valve, *43*, 44
APTT. *See* Activated partial thromboplastin
  time (APTT)
Arterial puncture(s), equipment for, 87
  procedures for, 87-89, *88*
Arteriole(s), 48
Artery(ies). *See also* names of specific arteries
  anatomy of, 45-46, *46*
  blood circulation through body, 46-48, *47*
ASCP. *See* American Society of Clinical Pathol-
  ogists (ASCP)
ASPT. *See* American Society of Phlebotomy
  Technicians (ASPT)
Atrioventricular (AV) node, 42-43, *44*
Atrium(a), defined, 41, *43*
Autolet skin puncture device, 59, *59*
AV bundle, 42-43, *44*

Biosafety techniques. *See* Infection prevention;
  Safety
Bleeding time, as platelet activity test, 49
  phlebotomy procedure for, 111-113,
    111-113

preparation of patient for, 110
purpose of, 110
values for, 113
Blood, amount of, in adult, 38
  circulation through body, 46-48, *47*
  circulation through heart, 41-45, *43-45*
  composition of, 38, *39*, 40-41, *40-42*
  history of diagnostic examination of, 1
  instruments of obtaining, history of, 1-4, *2-4*
  maximum amount to be drawn from pa-
    tients under 14 years of age, *79*
  viscosity of, conditions affecting, 96
Blood collection. *See also* Arterial puncture(s);
  Venipuncture
  bleeding time, 110-113, *111-113*
  blood cultures, 104, *105*, 106
  cold agglutinins, 109
  crossmatches, 102-104
  fibrin degradation products, 109-110
  general requirements for, 115-118
  heparin lock procedure, 113-114
  identification of patient for, 103
  oral glucose tolerance test (GTT), 106, *107*,
    108-109, *108*
  special techniques for, 102-114
Blood collection system, additives in, and their
  action, 64
  anticoagulant action and, 62, *62*, 64
  diagrams of equipment, 52-61, *53-62*
  disposable blood lancets, 58-59, *58*, *59*
  evacuated, 52, *53*, *54*, 65-67, 68, *69*, 80-81,
    80
  microtainer, 60, *60*
  Monovette system, 57, *57*
  nonevacuated, 52-53, *55*, *56*
  safety devices for, 67-68, *67*, *68*
  Sarstedt capillary blood collection system,
    61, *61*, *62*
  spring-loaded skin puncture devices, 59, *59*
  StatSampler, 60, *60*
  stopper color coding for, 63
  troubleshooting for the evacuated blood col-
    lection system, 65-67
  tube and holder size for evacuated system,
    68, *69*

123

UNOPETTE System, 61, *61*
Blood culture(s), history of, 1-2
  phlebotomy procedure for, 104, *105*, 106
  preparation of patient for, 104
  purpose of, 104
  values for, 106
Blood lancet(s), disposable, 58-59, *58*, *59*
Blood smear, coverslip procedure, 92-93, *93*
  preparation of, 92-96, *93-95*
  slide wedge procedure, 93-96, *94*, *95*
Blood specimen(s), procedure when unable to
    obtain, 90-91. *See also* Blood collection
Blood type, 102-103
Body Substance Isolation, as biosafety tech-
    nique, 14-15
Bundle of His, 42-43, *44*

Calcium, 62, 66-67
CAP. *See* College of American Pathologists
    (CAP)
Capillary(ies), *47*, 48
Cardiac muscle, defined, 45
CDC. *See* Centers for Disease Control (CDC)
Centers for Disease Control (CDC), 14
Certifying agencies, 4, 121-122
Children. *See also* Infants
  maximum amount of blood to be drawn
    from patients under 14 years of age,
    79
  refusal of venipuncture, 90-91
Circulation, history of, 4-6, *5-6*
  physiology of, 45-46, *46*
  through body, 46-48, *47*
  through heart, 41-45, *43-45*
Clotting. *See* Coagulation
Coagulation, cascade concept of, *49*, 50
  definition of, 48
  description of, 48-50, *48*, *49*
  disseminated   intravascular   coagulation,
    109-110
  fibrin degradation products, 109-110
  platelets and, 48-49
Coagulation factors, 49
Code of ethics, of American Society for Medi-
    cal Technology, 8
Cold agglutinin(s), phlebotomy procedure for,
    109
  purpose of, 109
  values for, 109
College of American Pathologists (CAP), 10
Color coding, for blood collection system, 63
Communication, importance of, 22
Contact transmission, of infectious disease
    agents, 13
Coronary artery(ies), 45
Coverslip procedure, for preparation of blood
    smear, 92-93, *93*
Crossmatch(es), phlebotomy procedure for,
    103-104

purpose of, 102-103
Culture, of blood. *See* Blood culture

Definitions, of medical terms, 24-31
DIC. *See* Disseminated intravascular coagula-
    tion (DIC)
Disseminated intravascular coagulation (DIC),
    109-110
Duke method, for determining bleeding time,
    113

Educational material, sources of, 119-120
Elastin, defined, 46, *46*
Endocarditis, defined, 41
Endocardium, defined, 41
Erythrocyte(s), 38, *39*, 40, *40*, *41*
Ethics, 7-8
Evacuated blood collection system, diagrams
    of equipment, 52, *53*, *54*
  history of, 2, 4, *4*
  order of draw for, 80-81, *80*
  troubleshooting for, 65-67
  tube and holder size for, 68, *69*

Fabricius of Aquapendente, and circulation, 6
FDP. *See* Fibrin degradation product(s) (FDP)
"Female-Luer," 52-53, *56*
Fibrin, blood composition and, 38
Fibrin clot, 49
Fibrin degradation product(s) (FDP), descrip-
    tion of, 109-110
  phlebotomy procedure for, 110
  purpose of, 110
Fibrinogen, and blood composition, 38
Fibrinolysis, 50, 109, 110
Finger stick, 83, *84*
FloTop Collector, 60, *60*

Galen, on circulation, 5, *5*
Gloving. *See* Gowning, gloving, masking
Glucose tolerance curve, 108-109, *108*
Glucose tolerance test (GTT), calculator for,
    106, *107*
  phlebotomy procedure for, 106, *107*, 108-
    109, *108*
  preparation of patient for, 106
  purpose of, 106
Gowning, gloving, masking, as safety proce-
    dure, 14-15
  technique for, 17-21, *17-21*
GTT. *See* Glucose tolerance test (GTT)

Handwashing, as safety procedure, 11, 14
  technique for, 15-17, *15-17*
Harvey, William, on circulation, 6, *6*
Heart, anatomy and physiology of, 41-45,
    43-45
  and circulation, description of, 38-50
  cardiac cycle, 44, *45*

conduction system of, 42-43, *44*
 weight of, 45
"Heart attack," description of, 45
Heel stick, on infant, 83, *83, 84*
Hemalet skin puncture device, 59, *59*
Hemostasis, primary, 48
 secondary, 49
 tests for evaluation of, 49
Heparin lock procedure, equipment for, 113-114
 phlebotomy procedure for, 114
Hepatitis A virus, 13
Hepatitis B virus, 10, 14
Hepatitis C virus, 13
Hippocrates, on circulation, 4
HIV. *See* Human immunodeficiency virus (HIV)
Human immunodeficiency virus (HIV), 13, 14
Hwang-Ti, on circulation, 4

Infant(s), heel stick on, 83, *83, 84*
 nursery technique, 10
Infection prevention, biosafety techniques, 14-21, *15-21*
 Body Substance Isolation, 14-15
 transmittal of infectious disease agents, 13-14
 universal precautions, 14-15
Infectious disease agents, airborne or inhalation transmission of, 13
 contact transmission of, 13
 ingestion transmission of, 13-14
 transmittal of, 13-14
 vectorborne transmission of, 14
Inferior vena cava, 48
Ingestion transmission, of infectious disease agents, 13-14
Inhalation transmission, of infectious disease agents, 13

JCAHO. *See* Joint Commission on Accreditation of Healthcare Organizations (JCAHO)
Joint Commission on Accreditation of Healthcare Organizations (JCAHO), 10

Keidel vacuum tube, and history of phlebotomy, 4, *4*
Ktesibios, and piston-and-cylinder syringe, 1, *2*

Laboratory tests. *See also* names of specific tests
 abbreviations for, 35-37
 clinical usefulness of, 35-37
 special instructions for, 115-118
Lancet(s), disposable blood lancets, 58-59, *58, 59*
 history of, *3*
 Safety Flow Lancet, 58, *58*

Tenderfoot, 58, *58*
Tenderlett, 59, *59*
Luer, in nonevacuated blood collection system, 52-53, *55, 56*

"Male-Luer," 52-53, *56*
Malpighi, Marcello, on circulation, 6
Manual of Clinical Diagnosis, and history of phlebotomy, 1-2
Marrow, red cell distribution of, *40*
Masking. *See* Gowning, gloving, masking
Medical terms and abbreviations, 22-37
Microtainer, 60, *60*
Mitral valve, *43*, 44
Monoject Safety Syringe, 68, *68*
Monojector skin puncture device, 59, *59*
Monovette system, 57, *57*
Myocardial infarction, defined, 45
Myocardium, defined, 45

National Certification Agency for Medical Laboratory Personnel (NCA), 4, 122
National Phlebotomy Association (NPA), 4, 122
NCA. *See* National Certification Agency for Medical Laboratory Personnel (NCA)
Nonevacuated blood collection system, 52-53, *55, 56*
NPA. *See* National Phlebotomy Association (NPA)
Nursery technique, 10

Occupational Safety and Health Administration (OSHA), 10
Oral glucose tolerance test (GTT), 106, *107*, 108-109, *108*
OSHA. *See* Occupational Safety and Health Administration (OSHA)

Pericarditis, defined, 41
Pericardium, defined, 41
Phlebotomy, certifying agencies in, 4, 121-122
 educational materials for, 119-120
 history of, 1-6, *2-6*
 national organizations in, 4
 professionalism in, 7-8
Plasma, description of, 38, *39. See also* Blood
Plasmin, 50, 109
Plasminogen, 50
Platelet(s), coagulation and, 48-49
 description of, 38, *39*, 41, 48, *48*
Platelet activity, primary tests for, 49
Platelet count, 49
Polycythemia, 96
Praxagoras of Cos, on circulation, 4-5
Prefix(es), suffix(es), and root word(s), 23-24
Prenatal screen, 102
Professionalism, and code of ethics, 7-8
 definition of, 7

personal appearance and, 8
Pro-Ject, 68, *68*
Prothrombin time (PT), 50
PT. *See* Prothrombin time (PT)
Pulmonary artery, *43*, 44, 47, *47*
Pulmonary valve, *43*, 44
Pulmonary vein(s), *43*, 44, 47, *47*
Purkinje fiber(s), 42-43, *44*

Red blood cell(s), description of, 38, *39*, 40, *40*, *41*
Rh factor, 102
Root word(s), prefix(es), and suffix(es), 23-24

Safety, biosafety techniques, 14-21, *15-21*
    blood collection system safety devices, 67-68, *67*, *68*
    Body Substance Isolation, 14-15
    general rules for, 10-12
    personal appearance and, 10
    universal precautions, 14-15
Safety Flow Lancet, 58, *58*
Saf-T Clik, 67-68, *67*
Sarstedt capillary blood collection system, *62*
Screen, for surgical patients, 103
Serum, description of, 38, *39. See also* Blood
Servetus, Michael, 5
Shamrock Safety Blood Collection Set, 68, *68*
Sinoatrial (SA) node, 42-43, *44*
Skin puncture, equipment for, 59, *59*, 82
    finger stick, 83, *84*
    heel stick, on infant, 83, *83*, *84*
    principle of, 82
    procedure for, 82-85, *83*, *84*
    quality assurance, 85
Skin puncture device(s), Autolet, 59, *59*
    Hemalet, 59, *59*
    Monojector, 59, *59*
    spring-loaded, 59, *59*
Slide wedge procedure, for preparation of blood smear, 92-93, *95*
StatSampler, 60, *60*
Suffix(es), prefix(es), and root word(s), 23-24
Superior vena cava, 48
Surgical patients, screen for, 103
Symbols, meanings of, 35
Syringe(s), for nonevacuated blood collection system, 52-53, *55*, *56*
    Monoject Safety Syringe, 68, *68*
    piston-and-cylinder, history of, 1, *2*

Tenderfoot lancet, 58, *58*
Tenderlett lancet, 59, *59*
Thrombin, 67, 109, 110
Todd, James C., and history of phlebotomy, 1-2

Tourniquet, application of, 73, *73-75*, 75
Troubleshooting, for the evacuated blood collection system, 65-67
Tunica externa (adventitia), 46, *46*
Tunica interna (intima), 45-46, *46*
Type and Rh, 102
Type and screen, 103

Universal precautions, as biosafety technique, 14-15
UNOPETTE Brand hematology system, components of, *98*
    description of, 97
    equipment for, 61, *61*
    manual white blood cell count of, 97-101, *98-101*
    procedure for, 97-101, *98-101*

VACUTAINER Brand, 2, 4
Value(s), for bleeding time, 113
    for blood cultures, 106
    for cold agglutinins, 109
Vectorborne transmission, of infectious disease agents, 14
Vein(s). *See also* names of specific veins
    anatomy of, 45-46, *46*
    blood circulation through body, 46-48, *47*
    selection of, for venipuncture, 73-75, *73-76*
Vena cava, superior and inferior, 48
Venipuncture, difficult, procedure for, 91
    patient not in room for, 90
    patient refusal of, 90-91
    procedure when unable to obtain blood specimens, 90-91
    routine, 71-81
        equipment for, 71
        maximum amount to be drawn from patients under 14 years of age, *79*
        most important step in, 71-72
        order of draw for evacuated blood collection system, 80-81, *80*
        principle of, 71
        procedure for, 71-78, *73-78*
        quality assurance, 78-81, *79*, *80*
    sites other than arms for, 91
Venous valve(s), defined, 46
Ventricle(s), defined, 41, *43*
Venule(s), defined, 48
Viscosity of blood, 96

White blood cell(s), 38, *39*, 42
White blood cell count, by UNOPETTE system, 97-101, *98-101*
White blood cell differential, history of, 1-2
Words and terms, definitions of, 24-31